Plant-Based Diet for Busy People

Quick and Easy Recipes to Enjoy Plant-Based Meals and Improve Your Health

I0145952

Clay Palmer

Table of Contents

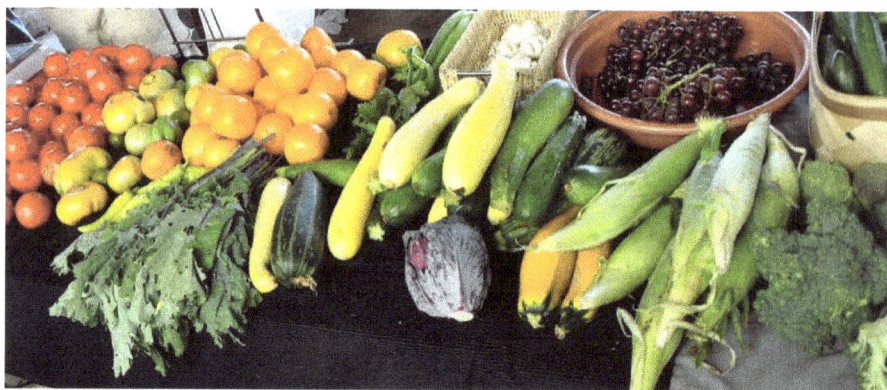

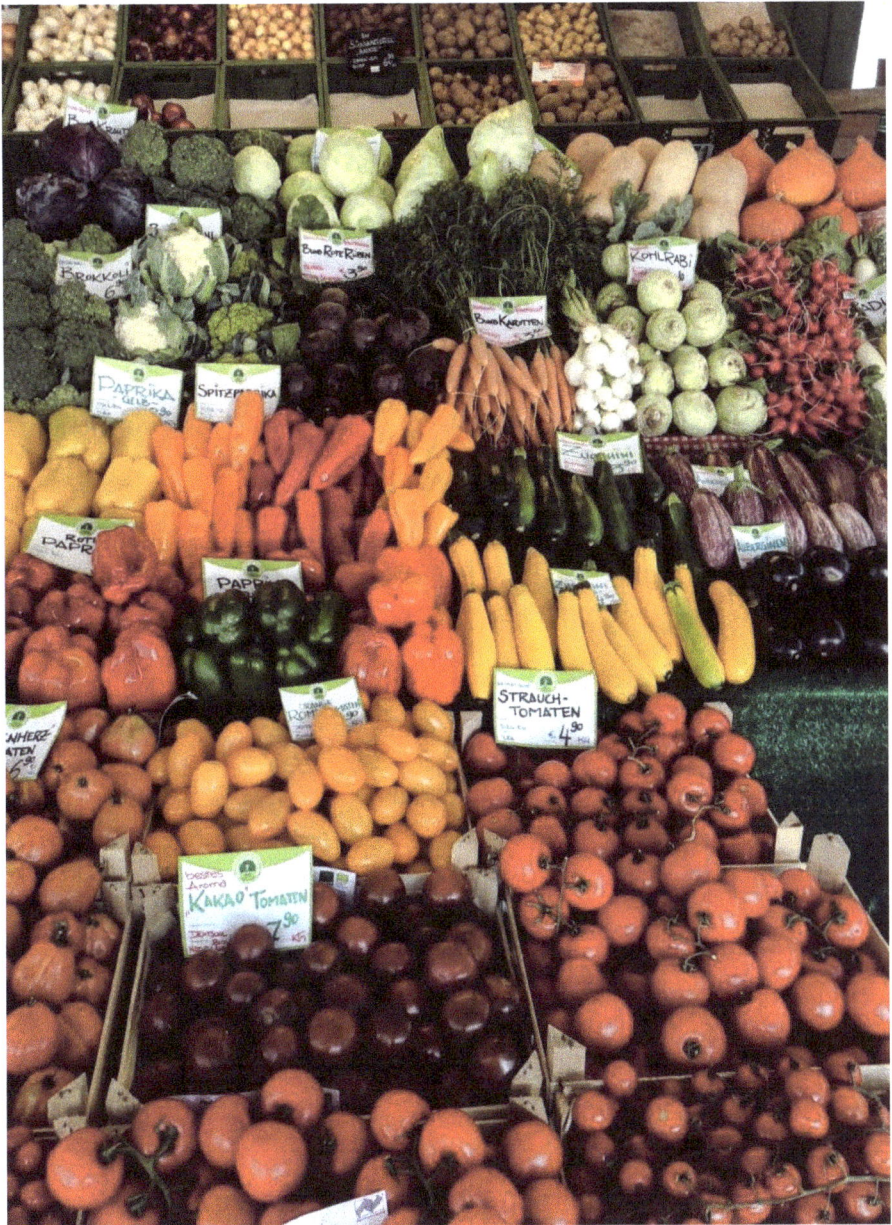

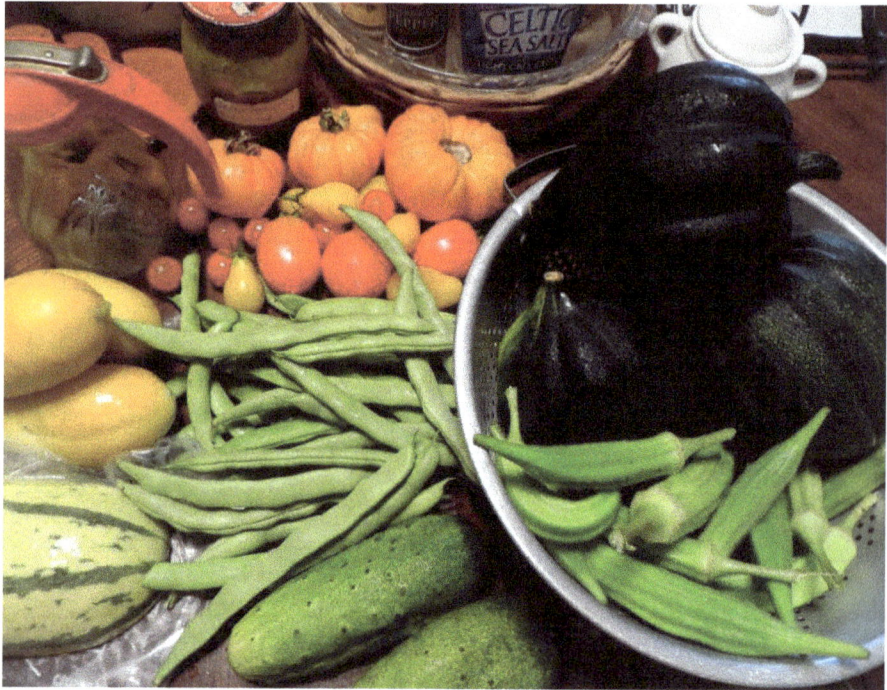

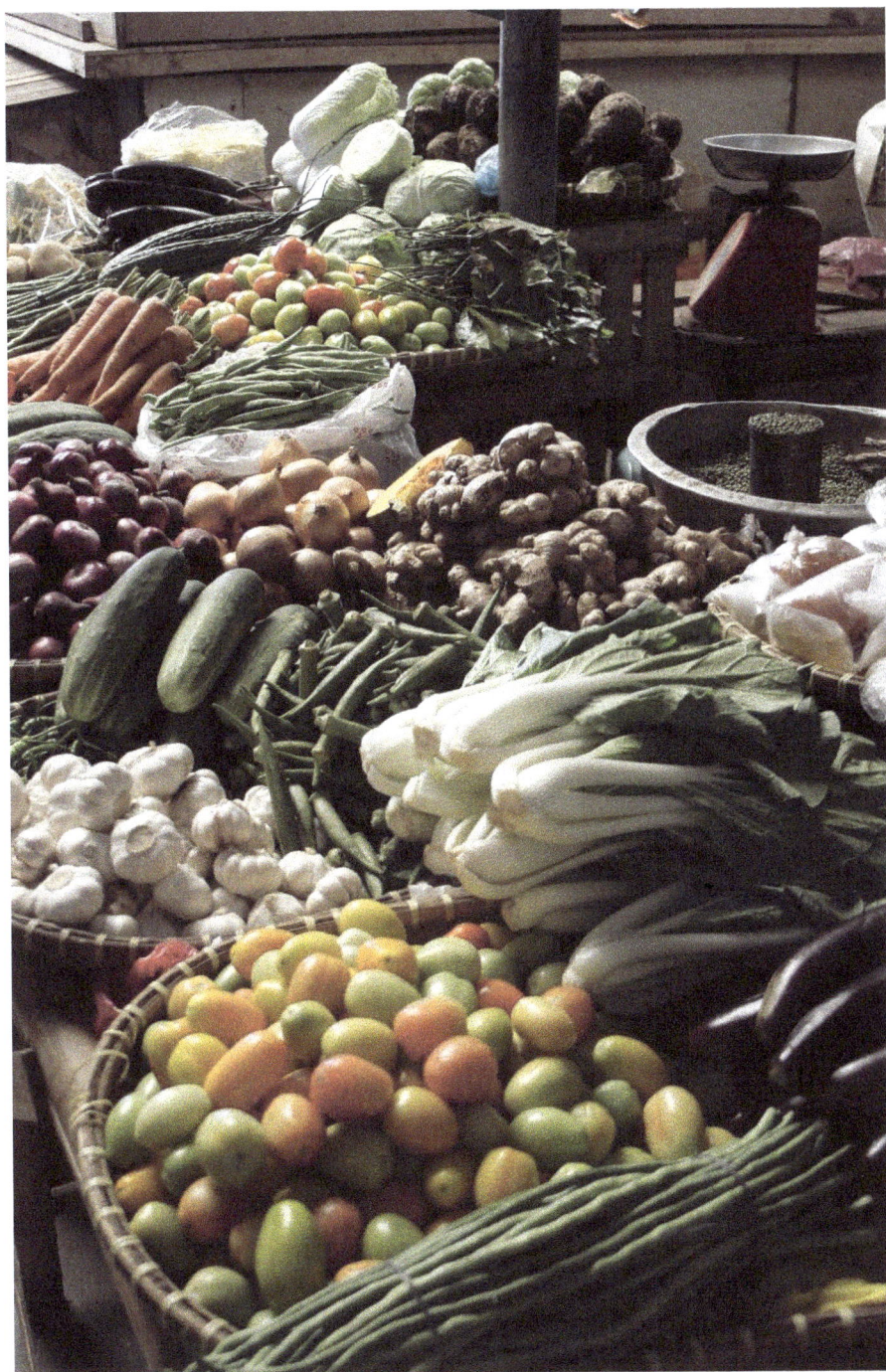

Stunning Steamed Asparagus

Preparation time: 10 minutes Cooking time: 30 minutesServings: 4.

Ingredients:

3 cups water 1 tsp. vegan butter 3 cups asparagus salt and pepper to taste

Directions:

Begin by pouring water into a steamer. Add the butter, and bring the water to a boil. Next, place the asparagus in the top of the steamer, and steam the asparagus for ten minutes. Enjoy warm with a bit of salt.

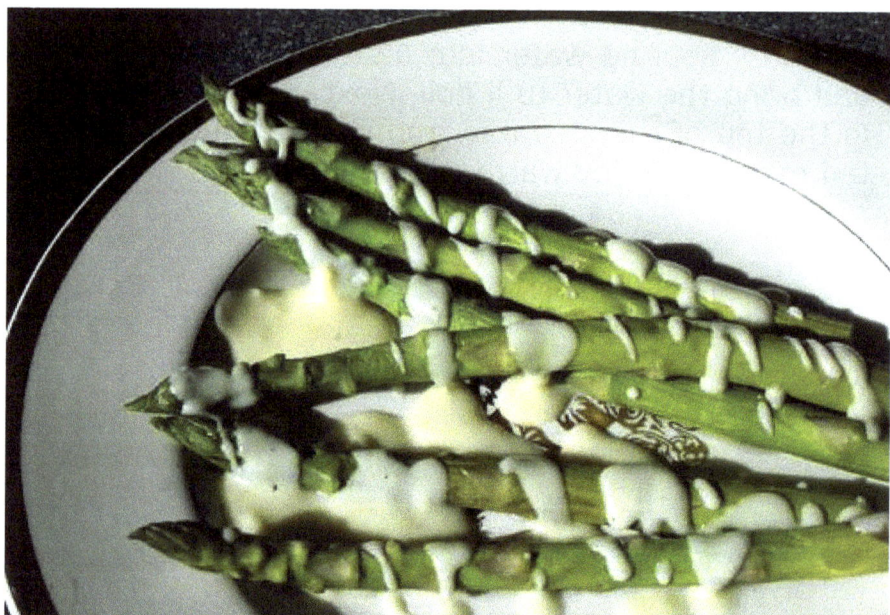

Electric Garlic Kale

Preparation time: 10 minutes Cooking time: 50 minutesServings: 4.

Ingredients:

3 cups kale 5 minced garlic cloves 3 tbsp. olive oil

Directions:

Begin by tearing up the kale leaves. Heat the olive oil in a skillet, and allow the garlic to heat in the olive oil for three minutes before adding the kale. Cook the kale for five minutes more, and serve warm.

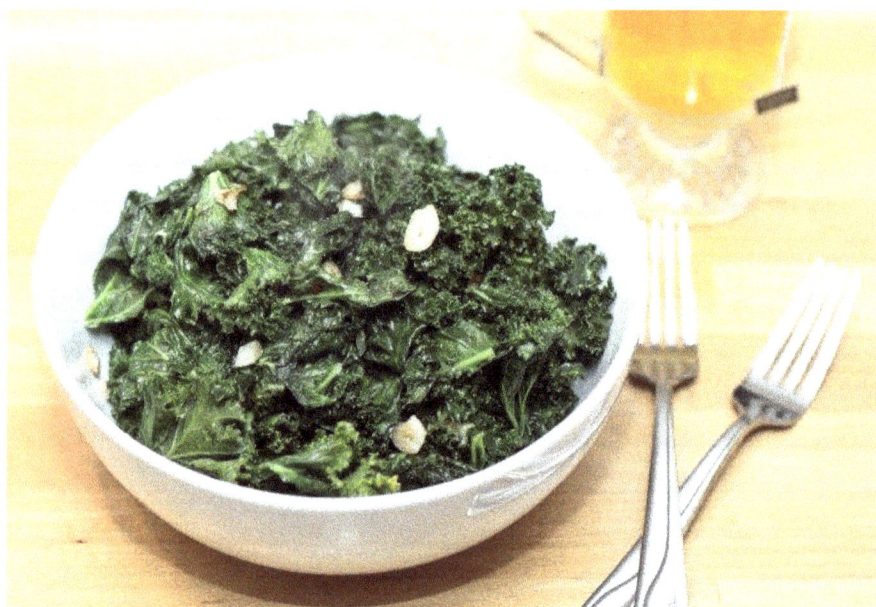

Super-Hot Red Cherry Tomatoes

Preparation time: 10 minutes Cooking time: 60 minutesServings: 4.

Ingredients:

1 tsp. sugar 2 tsp. vegan butter 2 tsp. basil 1 1/3 pint cherry tomatoes salt and pepper to taste

Directions:

Begin by melting the vegan butter in a skillet. Add the basil, the sugar, and the tomatoes to the skillet, and cook them for forty seconds. Season them with salt and pepper. Next, cook the tomatoes until the tomatoes begin to blacken, and then serve the tomatoes warm. Enjoy

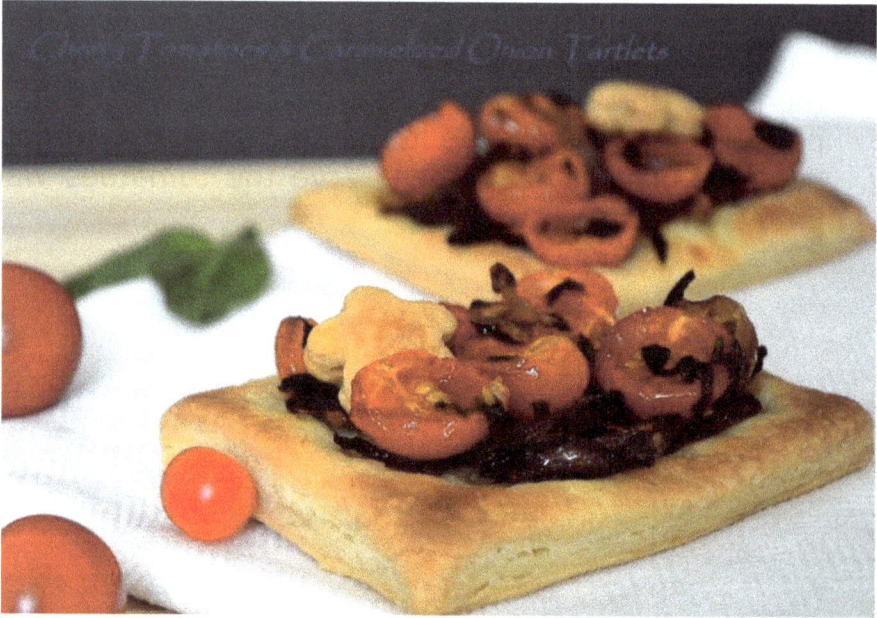

Cherry Tomatoes & Caramelized Onion Tartlets

Super-Sweet Sweet Potato Casserole

Preparation time: 10 minutes Cooking time: 40 minutesServings: 6.

Ingredients:

5 cups cubed sweet potatoes 2 egg substitutes ½ cup white sugar 4 tbsp. vegan butter 1 tsp. vanilla ½ cup soy milk Topping Ingredients: 1/3 cup brown sugar ¼ cup flour 4 tbsp. vegan butter 1/3 cup diced pecans

Directions:

Begin by preheating your oven to 325 degrees Fahrenheit. Next, pour the sweet potatoes in a saucepan with water. Allow the water to boil until the potatoes are tender. Next, mix together the sweet potatoes, the egg replacements, the sugar, the vegan butter, the soymilk, the vanilla, and the salt. Mix this together until completely smooth. Next, pour this mixture into a baking dish. To the side, mix together the brown sugar and the flour. Add the vegan butter (for the topping) and the pecans. Continue to stir, and sprinkle this mixture over the created baking dish mixture. Bake the sweet potatoes pie for thirty minutes. Enjoy warm.

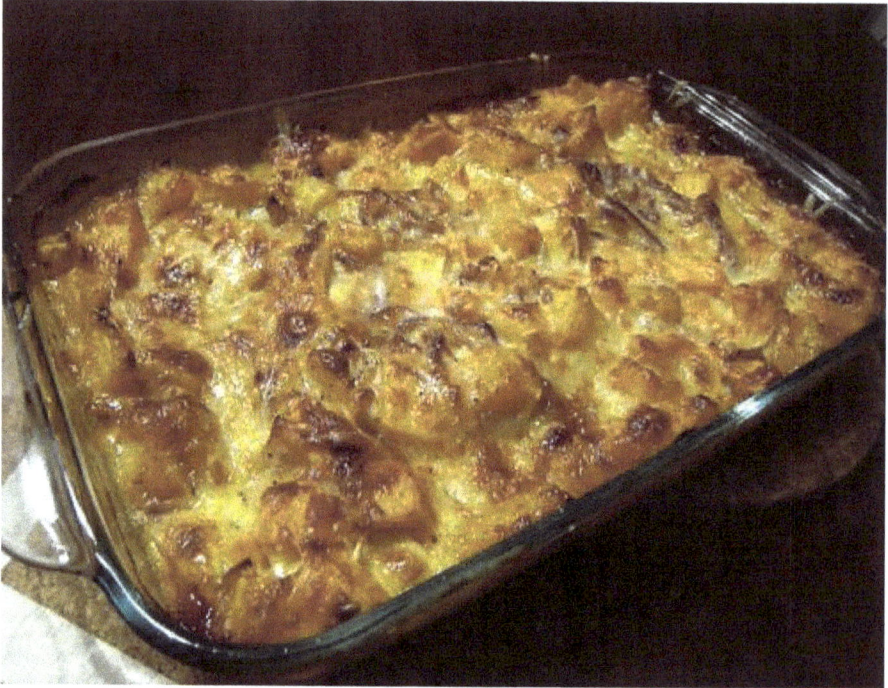

Zucchini Side Casserole

Preparation time: 10 minutes Cooking time: 40 minutesServings: 5.

Ingredients:

2 minced garlic cloves 1 sliced onion 2 pounds cubed zucchini 1 cup water ½ cup uncooked rice 3 tbsp. olive oil 2 tsp. garlic salt 2 cups chopped tomatoes 1 tsp. oregano 1 tsp. paprika 2 cups shredded vegan cheddar cheese

Directions:

Begin by mixing together the rice and the water in a saucepan and allowing it to simmer for twenty-five minutes. Next, preheat your oven to 350 degrees Fahrenheit. Pour the oil in a skillet and cook the onions, the zucchini, and the garlic for five minutes. Add all the seasoning, and then add the tomatoes, the rice, and the vegan cheese. Cook and stir continuously for five more minutes. Pour this mixture into a baking dish, and bake the casserole for twenty minutes. Enjoy!

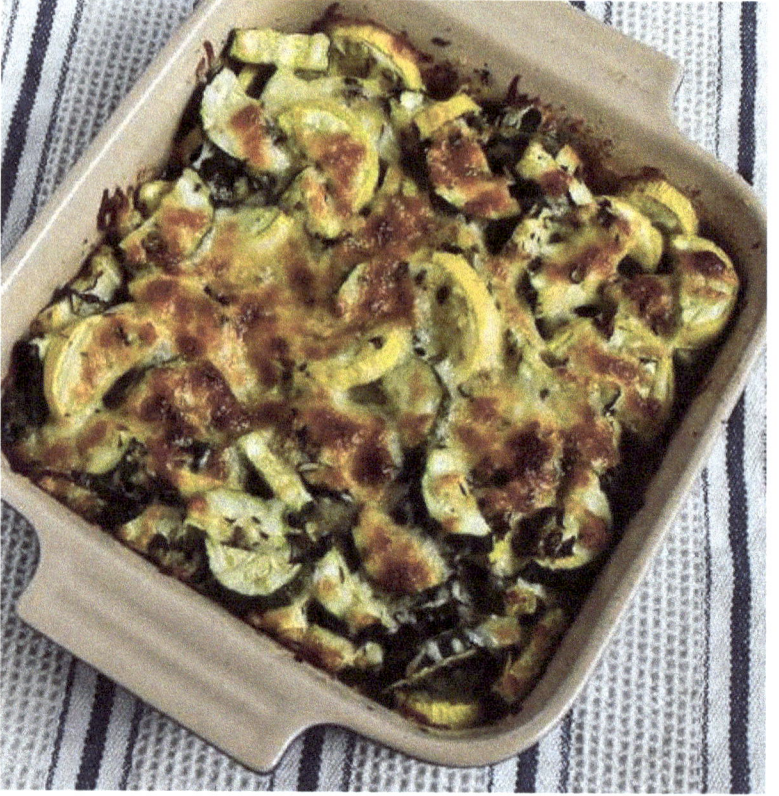

To the Side Roasted Butternut Squash

Preparation time: 10 minutes Cooking time: 30 minutesServings: 5.

Ingredients:

2 minced garlic cloves 3 cups peeled and cubed butternut squash 3 tbsp. olive oil salt and pepper to taste

Directions:

Begin by preheating the oven to 350 degrees Fahrenheit. Next, place the squash, the garlic, and the olive oil together in a large boil. Toss the squash, and then pour the squash into a baking sheet. Cook the squash for thirty minutes in the oven, and serve warm. Enjoy.

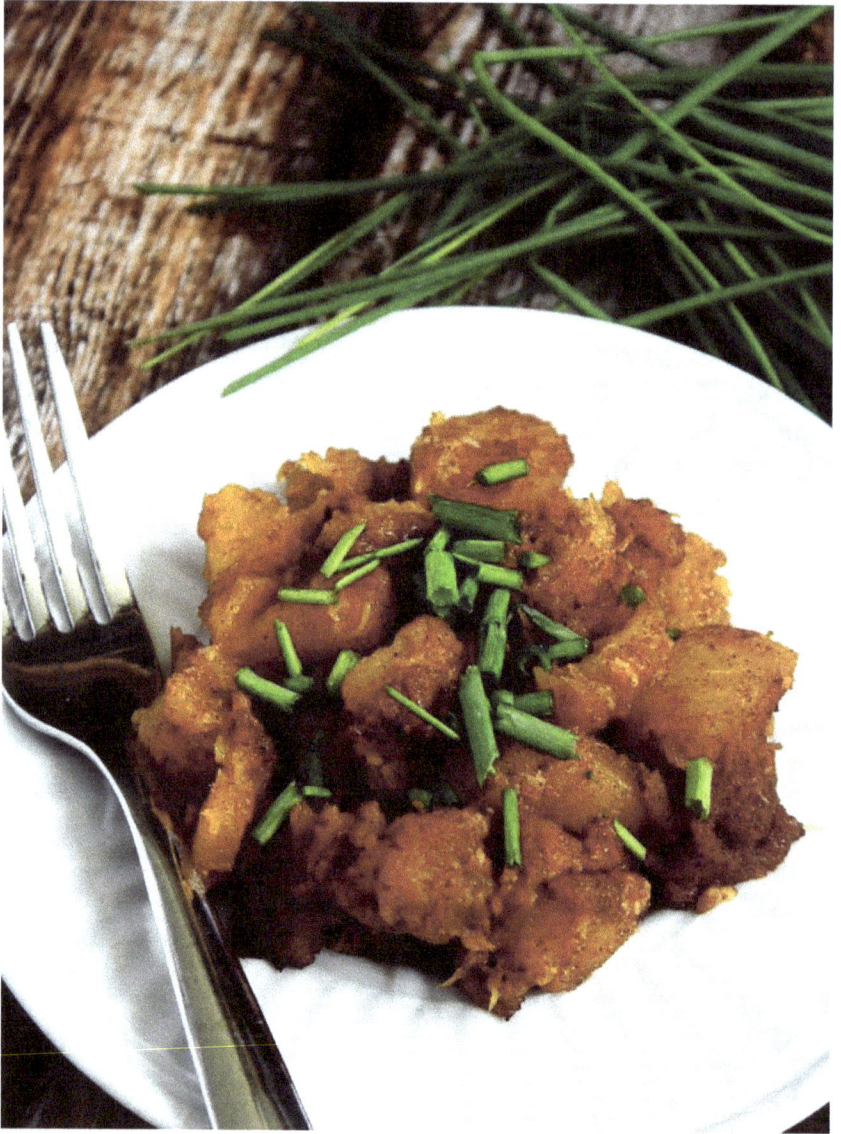

Beautiful Table Acorn Squash

Preparation time: 10 minutes Cooking time: 50 minutesServings: 2.

Ingredients:

1 halved and de-seeded acorn squash 5 tbsp. vegan butter 4 tbsp. brown sugar salt and pepper to taste

Directions:

Begin by pouring a bit of water in a microwave safe dish. Place the two squashes face-down in the water, and pierce the squash skin all over with a fork. Microwave the squash on high for twenty minutes, and then drain the casserole dish. Next, salt and pepper the squash, and portion out the butter and the brown sugar in each squash half. Broil the squash halved for five minutes, and the enjoy warm.

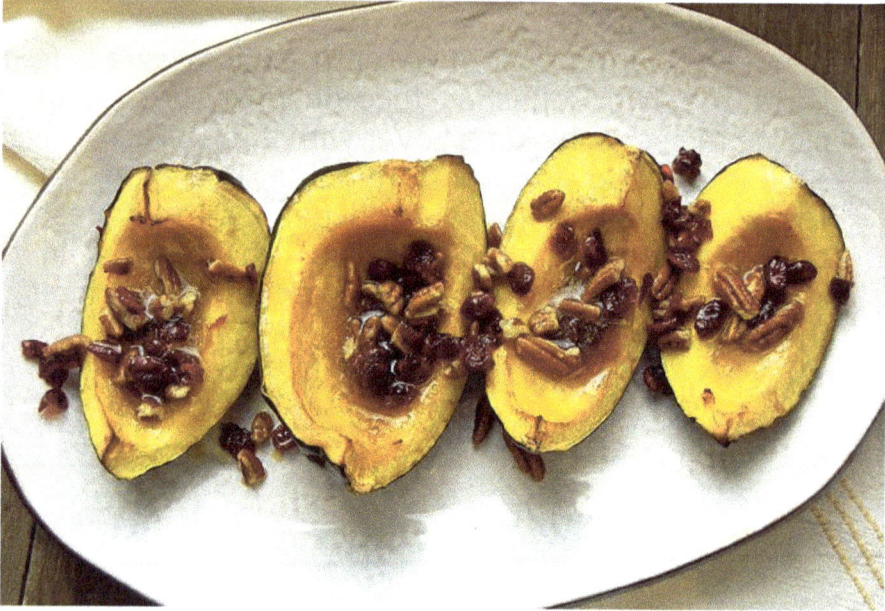

Fried Green Zucchini

Preparation time: 10 minutes Cooking time: 30 minutesServings: 4.

Ingredients:

2 sliced zucchinis 1 sliced onion 1/3 cup cornmeal ½ cup all-purpose flour ½ tsp. garlic powder 1 cup olive oil salt and pepper to taste

Directions:

Begin by placing the onions and the zucchini together in a medium-sized bowl. To the side, mix together the cornmeal, the flour, the garlic powder, and the salt and pepper. Pour this dry mix over the zucchini, and shake the mixture well. Allow the zucchini to sit for thirty minutes. Next, heat the olive oil over medium-high heat in a skillet. After the oil become shot, add the vegetables to the skillet and brown the vegetables evenly on all sides. Enjoy.

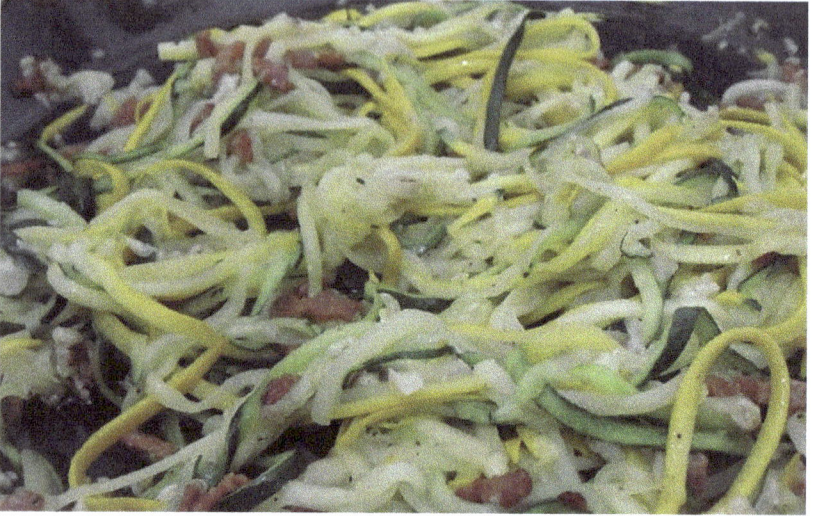

Beans and Greens

Preparation time: 10 minutes Cooking time: 60 minutesServings: 2.

Ingredients:

2 tbsp. olive oil 3 cups kale 2 cups beet greens 15 ounces cannelilini beans 3 minced garlic cloves 1 diced onion

Directions:

Begin by heating the olive oil, the onion, and the garlic in a skillet for five minutes. Next, add the greens and cover the pan, leaving an inch of air. Allow the greens to wilt, Next, add the beans and cook the mixture for five more minutes. Serve warm, and enjoy.

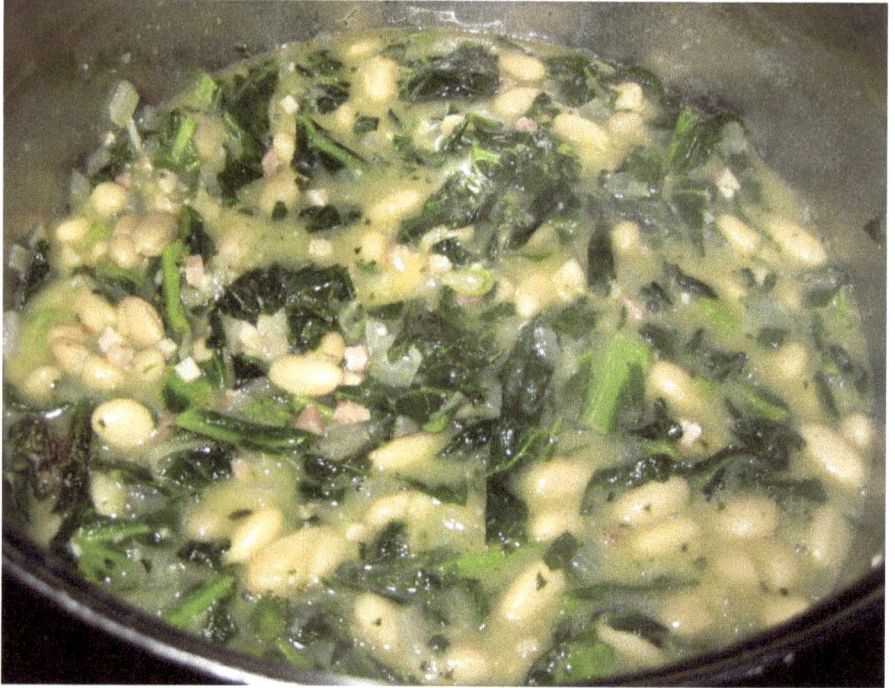

Creamy Tofu Spinach

Preparation time: 10 minutes Cooking time: 30 minutesServings: 8.

Ingredients:

12 ounces firm tofu 1 tbsp. butter 1 diced onion ½ cup soymilk 1 tbsp. olive oil 1 cup vegan Parmesan cheese 3 minced garlic cloves 2 pounds chopped spinach

Directions:

Begin by heating the olive oil, the onion, and the garlic together in a skillet. Add the spinach and allow it to wilt. Next, mix together the vegan cheese, vegan milk, and tofu together in a blender. Blend until completely smooth. Next, add the tofu mixture to the spinach, and cook the mixture until it's warm. Serve and enjoy!

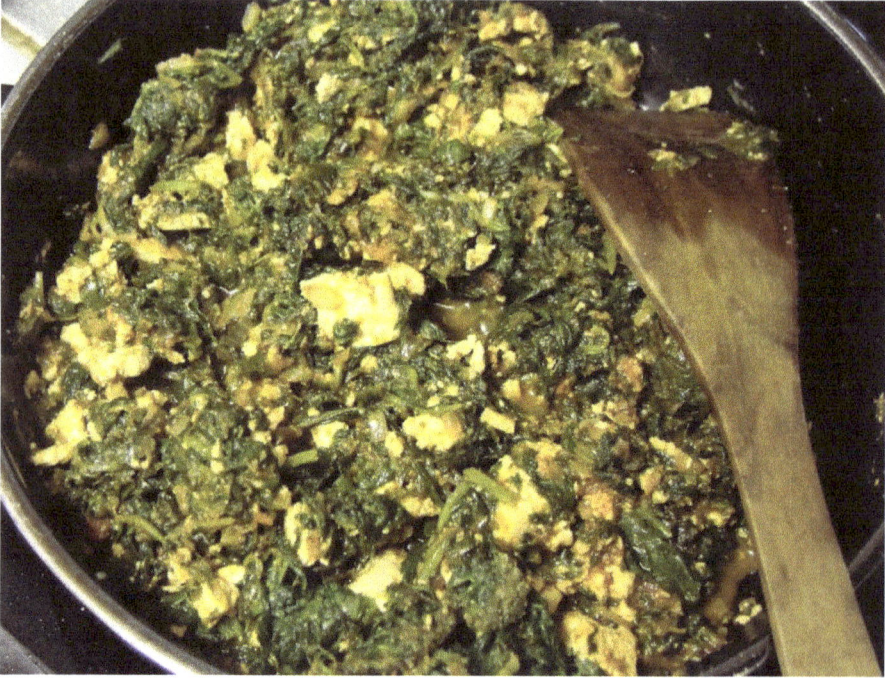

Summer Squash Mix

Preparation Time: 10 minutes Cooking Time: 1 Servings:

Ingredients

3 ounces coconut cream ½ teaspoon oregano, dried Salt and black pepper 1 big yellow summer squash, peeled and cubed 1/3 cup carrot, cubed 2 tablespoons olive oil

Directions:

In a pan that fits your Air Fryer, combine squash with carrot, oil, oregano, salt, pepper and coconut cream, toss, transfer to your Air Fryer and cook at 400 ° F for 10 minutes. Divide between plates and serve as a side dish.

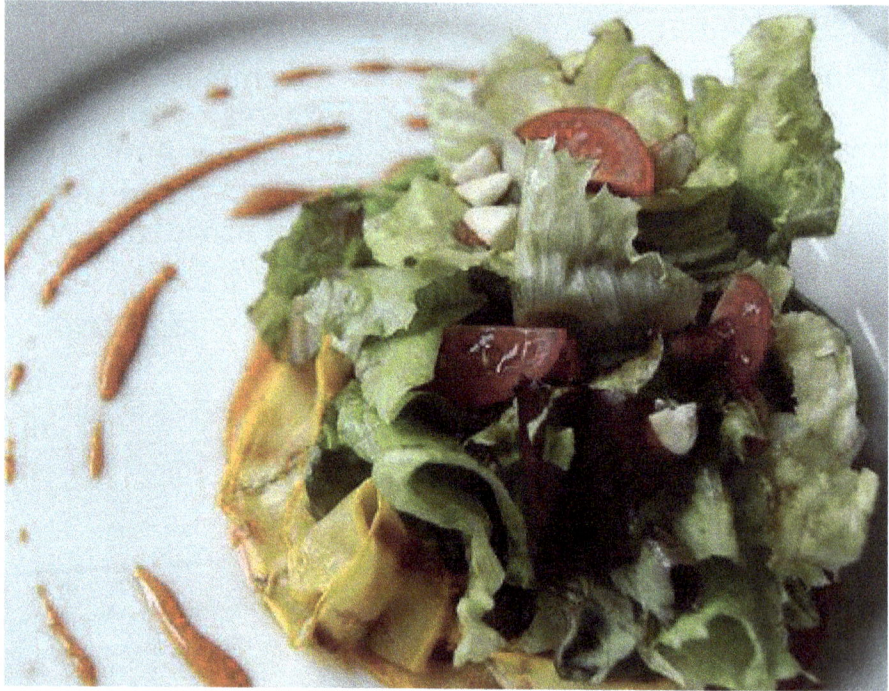

Baby Finger Burgers

Preparation time: 10 minutesCooking time: 45 minutes Servings: 4.

Ingredients:

15 ounce can of green lentils 2 tsp. paprika ½ tsp. garlic powder ¼ tsp. pepper 1 tbsp. tamari 1/3 cup wheat gluten 1 tsp. Worcestershire sauce 2 tbsp. olive oil 8 mini vegan buns 2 sliced dill pickles 8 toothpicks for skewering

Directions:

Begin by stirring together the paprika, the lentils, the garlic powder, the tamari, the pepper, and the Worcestershire sauce in a medium-sized bowl. Mash up the ingredients to make sure that most of the lentils are mashed. Next, stir in the wheat gluten and continue to smash. You should create a dough ball. Remove about a tbsp. of the prepared dough, and place this dough on a clean surface. Lay out all sixteen balls of dough and flatten each of the balls into a hamburger patty. Heat the olive oil in a skillet and place each patty in the skillet, frying each side for about five minutes. Assemble your tiny burgers by placing the burger in the buns and administering your favorite toppings. (I chose dill pickles.) When you're finished, skewer the hamburgers and serve them warm at your party. Enjoy!

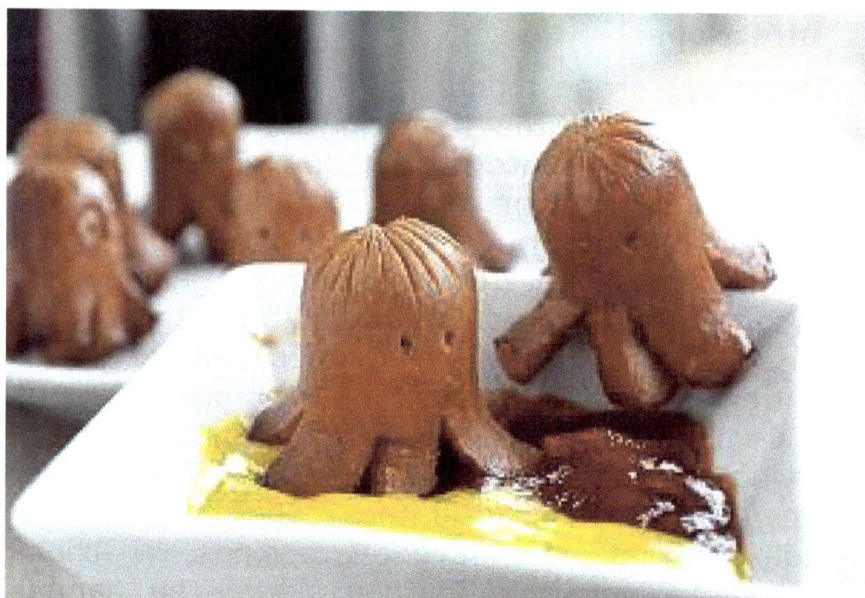

Broccoli, Tomatoes And Carrots

Preparation Time: 10 minutes Cooking Time: 14 minutes Servings:

Ingredients

1 broccoli head, florets separated and steamed 1 tomato, chopped 3 carrots, chopped and steamed 2 ounces soft tofu, crumbled 1 teaspoon parsley, chopped 1 teaspoon thyme, chopped Salt and black pepper to the taste

Directions:

In a pan that fits your Air Fryer, combine broccoli with tomato, carrots, thyme, parsley, salt and pepper, toss, introduce the fryer and cook at 350 ° F for 10 minutes. Add tofu, toss, introduce in the fryer for 4 minutes more, divide between plates and serve as a side dish.

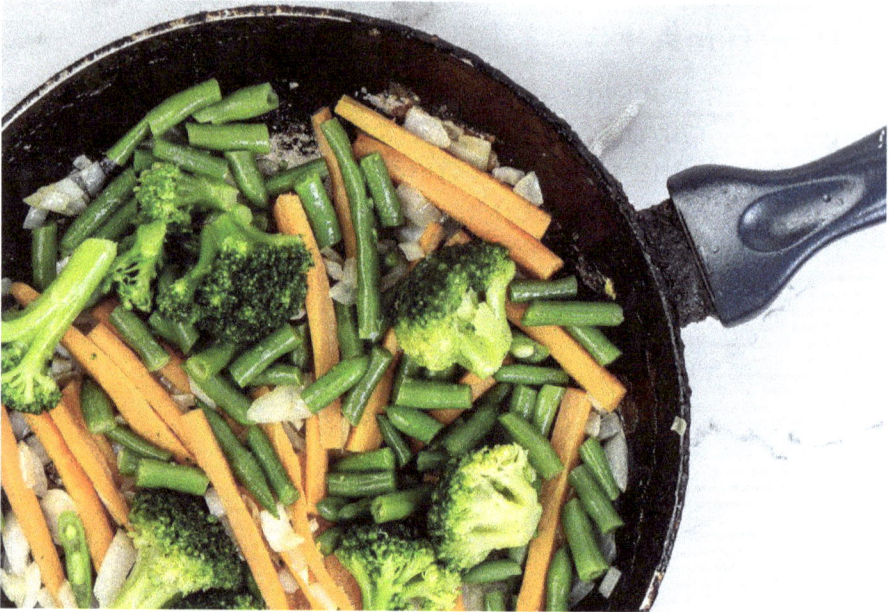

Mexican Black Beans

Preparation Time: 10 minutes Cooking time: 10 hours Servings: 4

Ingredients:

1 pound black beans, soaked overnight and drained A pinch of sea salt Black pepper to the taste 3 cups veggie stock 2 cups yellow onion, chopped 1 tablespoon canned chipotle chili pepper in adobo sauce 4 garlic cloves, minced 1 tablespoon lime juice ½ cup cilantro, chopped ½ cup pumpkin seeds

Directions:

Put the beans in your slow cooker. Add a pinch of salt, black pepper, onion, stock, garlic and chipotle chili in adobo sauce. Stir, cover and cook on Low for 10 hours. Add lime juice and mash beans a bit using a potato masher. Add cilantro, stir gently, divide between plates and serve with pumpkin seeds on top. Enjoy!

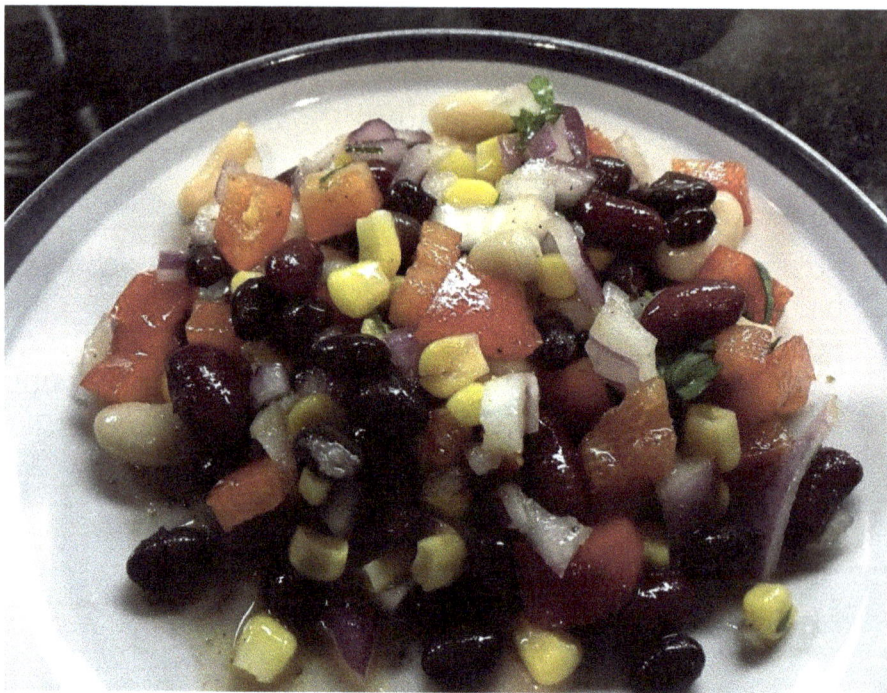

Summer Black Eyed Peas

Preparation Time: 10 minutes Cooking time: 8 hours Servings: 6

Ingredients:

3 cups black eyed peas A pinch of salt Black pepper to the taste 2 cups veggie stock 2 tablespoons jalapeno peppers, chopped 2 cups sweet onion, chopped ½ teaspoon thyme, dried 4 garlic cloves, minced 1 bay leaf Hot sauce to the taste

Directions:

Put the peas in your slow cooker. Add a pinch of salt, black pepper, stock, jalapenos, onion, garlic, thyme and bay leaf. Stir everything, cover and cook on Low for 8 hours. Drizzle hot sauce over peas, stir gently, divide between plates and serve. Enjoy!

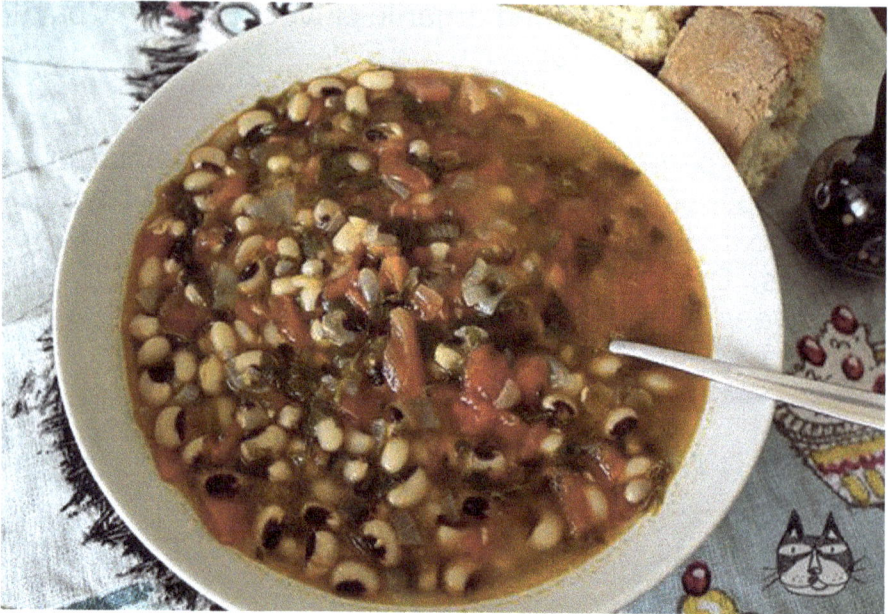

Great Beans and Lentils Dish

Preparation Time: 10 minutes Cooking time: 7 hours and 10 minutes Servings: 6

Ingredients:

2 tablespoons thyme, chopped 1 tablespoon olive oil 1 cup yellow onion, chopped 5 cups water 5 garlic cloves, minced 3 tablespoons cider vinegar ½ cup tomato paste ½ cup maple syrup 3 tablespoons soy sauce 2 tablespoons Korean red chili paste 2 tablespoons dry mustard 1 and ½ cups great northern beans ½ cup red lentils

Directions: Heat up a pan with the oil over medium high heat, add onion, stir and cook for 4 minutes. Add garlic, thyme, vinegar and tomato paste, stir, cook for 5 minutes more and transfer to your slow cooker. Add lentils and beans to your slow cooker and stir. Also add water, maple syrup, mustard, chili paste and soy sauce, stir, cover and cook on High for 7 hours. Stir beans mix again, divide between plates and serve. Enjoy!

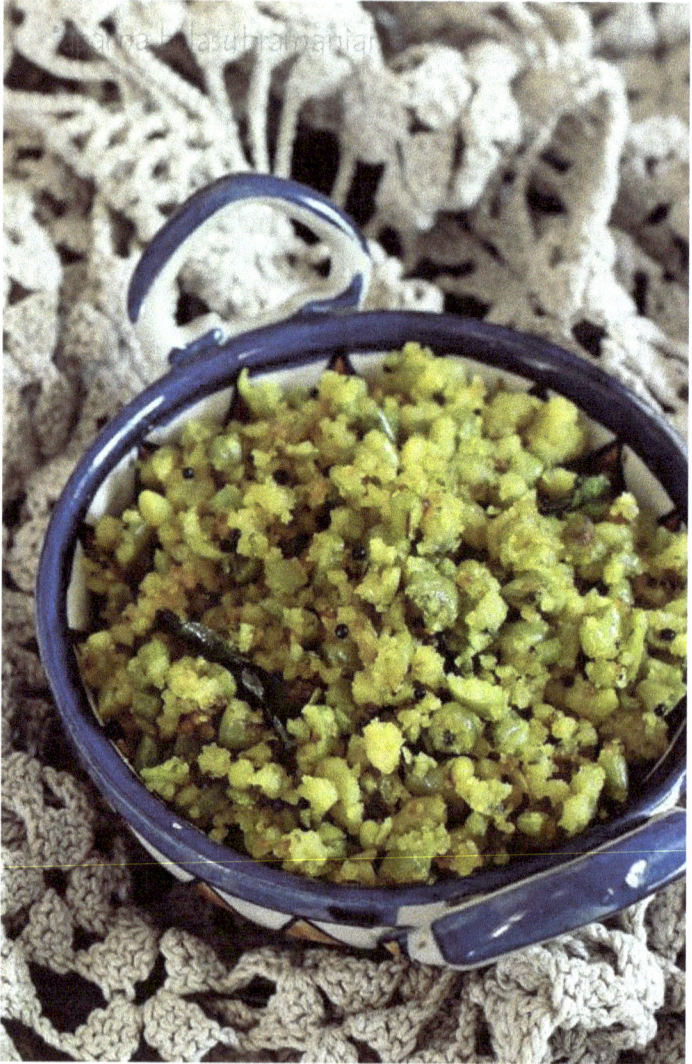

Wonderful Wild Rice

Preparation Time: 10 minutes Cooking time: 6 hours
Servings: 12

Ingredients:

42 ounces veggie stock 1 cup carrot, shredded 2 and ½ cups wild rice 4 ounces mushrooms, sliced 2 tablespoons olive oil 2 teaspoons marjoram, dried A pinch of sea salt Black pepper to the taste 2/3 cup cherries, dried ½ cup pecans, chopped 2/3 cup green onions, chopped

Directions:

Put the stock in your slow cooker. Add rice, carrots, mushrooms, oil, salt, pepper marjoram. Stir, cover and cook on Low for 6 hours. Add cherries and green onions, stir, cover slow cooker and leave it aside for 10 minutes. Divide wild rice between plates and serve with chopped pecans on top. Enjoy!

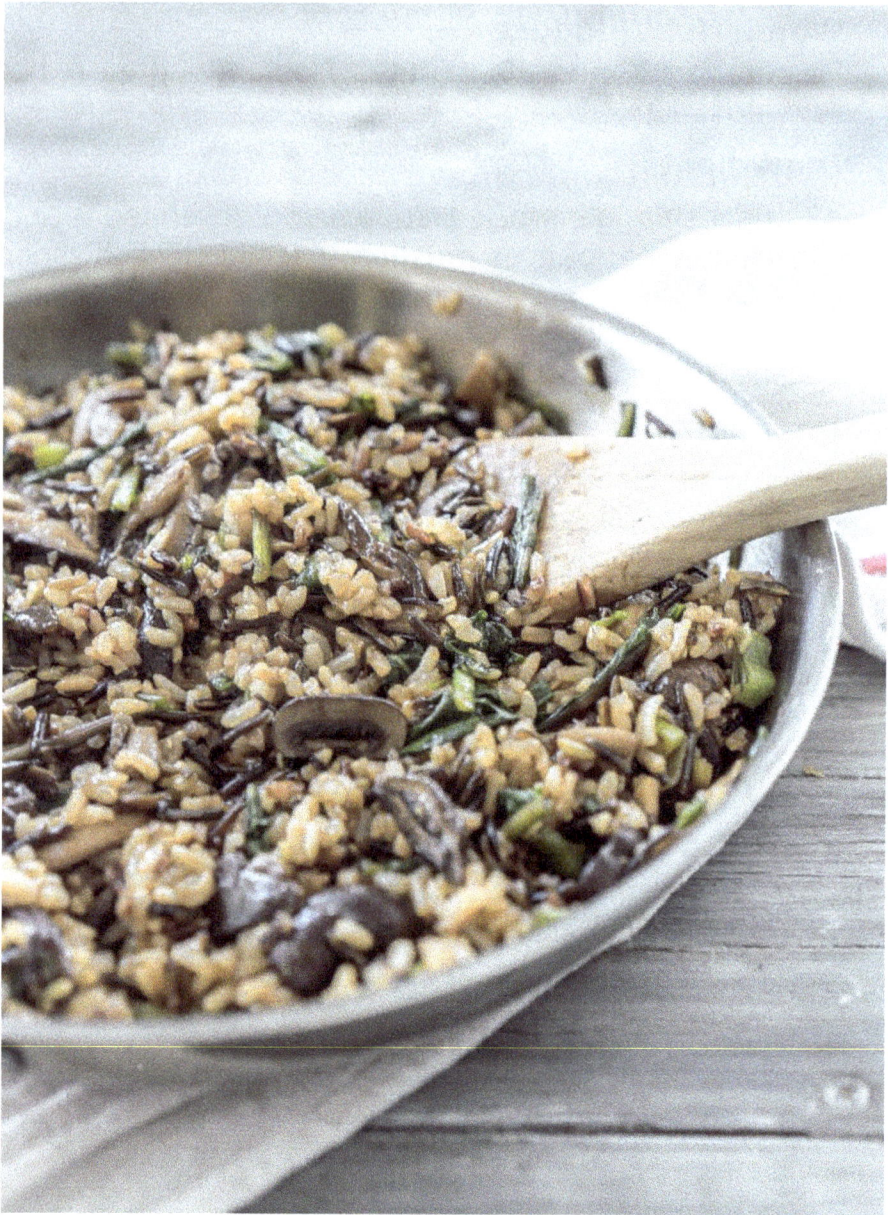

Delicious Barley and Squash Gratin

Preparation Time: 10 minutes Cooking time: 7 hours Servings: 12

Ingredients:

2 pounds butternut squash, peeled and cubed 1 yellow onion, cut into medium wedges 10 ounces spinach 1 cup barley 14 ounces veggie stock ½ cup water A pinch of salt Black pepper to the taste 3 garlic cloves, minced

Directions:

Put squash pieces in your slow cooker. Add barley, spinach, stock, water, onion, garlic, salt and pepper, stir, cover and cook on Low for 7 hours. Stir this mix again, divide between plates and serve. Enjoy!

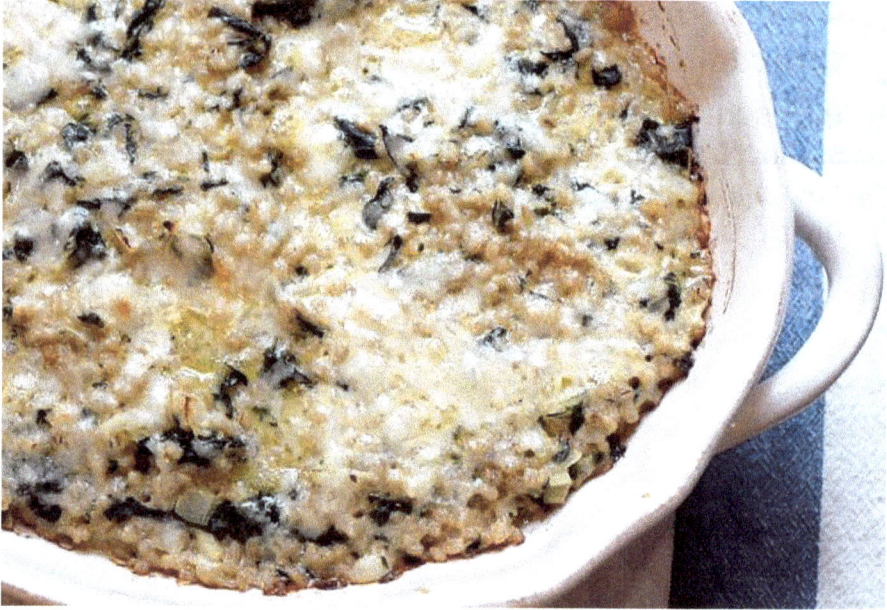

Thyme for Maple Syrup Sweet Potato Fries

Preparation time: 10 minutes Cooking time: 20 minutes Servings: 4.

Ingredients:

1 pound sliced sweet potatoes 1 sliced parsnip 1 sliced carrot 5 sprigs of thyme 3 tbsp. maple syrup olive oil

Directions:

Begin by preheating the oven to 375 degrees Fahrenheit. Next, place the sweet potatoes, the carrots, and the parsnips together over a jelly roll pan. Add the salt and pepper and the oil. Toss. Next, toss the ingredients into the oven and allow the vegetables to cook for thirty minutes. Place the thyme and the maple syrup over the vegetables, toss, and allow the vegetables to bake for twenty more minutes. Enjoy.

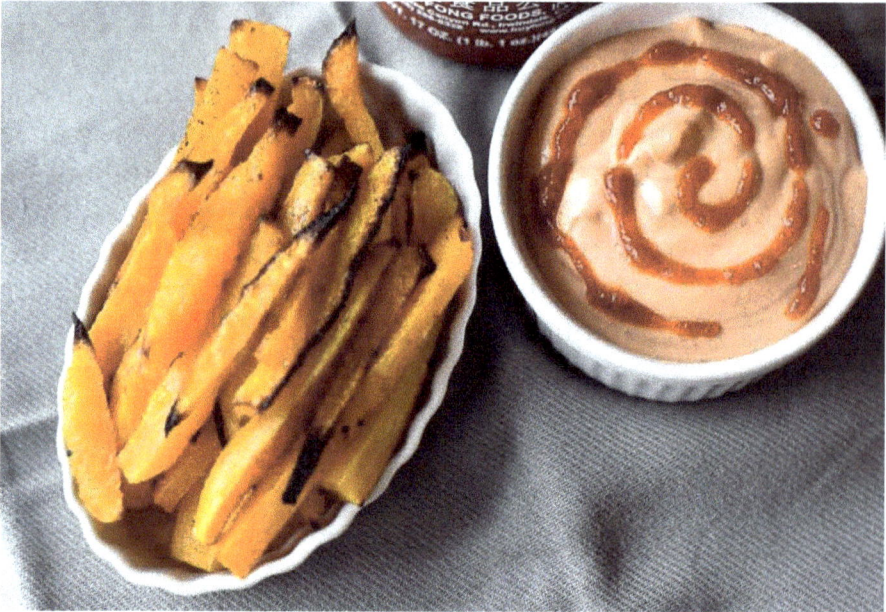

Super-Easy Applesauce

Preparation time: 10 minutes Cooking time: 35 minutesServings: 8.

Ingredients:

10 peeled and chopped apples 2 tsp. lemon juice ½ cup brown sugar 1 cup apple cider 2 tsp. cinnamon ½ tsp. salt

Directions:

Begin by mixing together the above ingredients in a large soup pot over medium. Allow the mixture to boil. Afterwards, allow the mixture to simmer for twenty-five minutes over low heat. Mash the ingredients with a potato masher, and serve the applesauce either warm or cold. Enjoy.

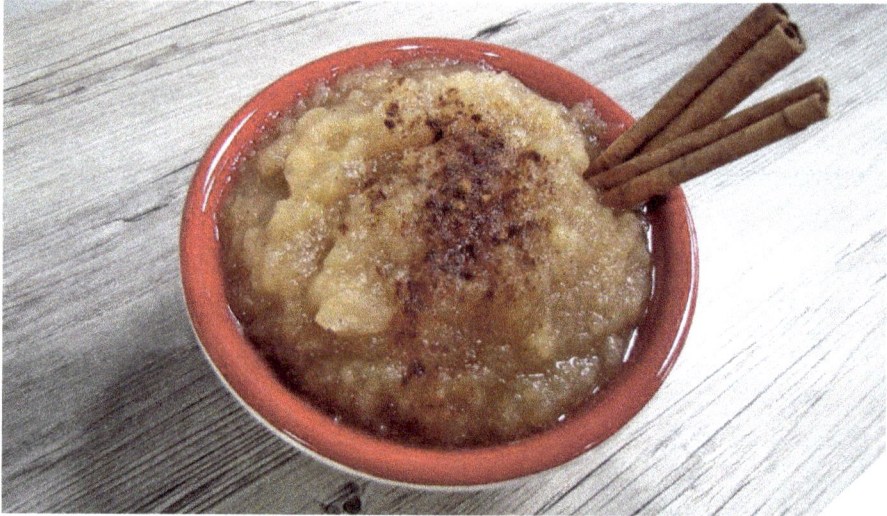

Primary Pear Applesauce

Preparation time: 10 minutes Cooking time: 30 minutesServings: 3.

Ingredients:

7 peeled and sliced apples 5 peeled and sliced pears ½ cup apple cider 2 ½ tbsp. cinnamon 1 ½ tbsp. sugar

Directions:

Begin by heating the apples, the pears, and the cider together in a large skillet for ten minutes. Next, smash the fruit together with a wooden smooth, and continue to cook the mixture for thirty minutes. Add the cinnamon and the sugar to the mixture at this time, stirring all the time, until it's completely cooked through—another ten minutes. Serve either warm or chilled, and enjoy!

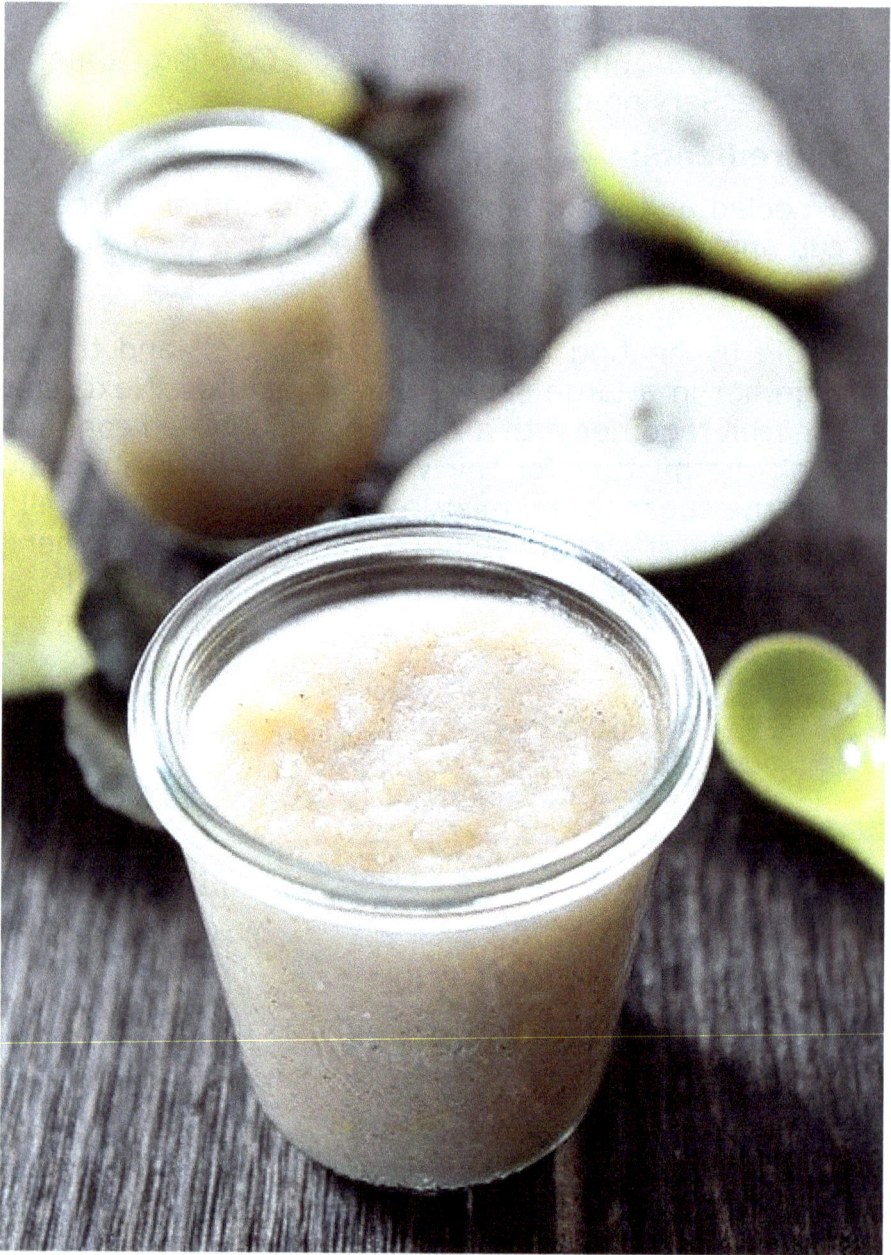

South of the Border Mexican Quinoa

Preparation time: 10 minutes Cooking time: 20 minutesServings: 4.

Ingredients:

10 ounces diced tomatoes 1 tbsp. olive oil 1 ½ cup quinoa 3 minced garlic cloves 1 diced onion 1 diced jalapeno pepper 2 cups vegetable broth 1/3 cup chopped cilantro 1 store-bought package taco seasoning

Directions:

Begin by heating the olive oil, the quinoa, and the onion in a skillet over high heat. Next, add the garlic and the jalapeno pepper, and cook the mixture for three minutes. Add the tomatoes, the seasoning, and the vegetable broth, and allow the mixture to boil. Place the heat on low, and allow it to simmer for twenty-five minutes. Next, add the cilantro, and serve warm. Enjoy.

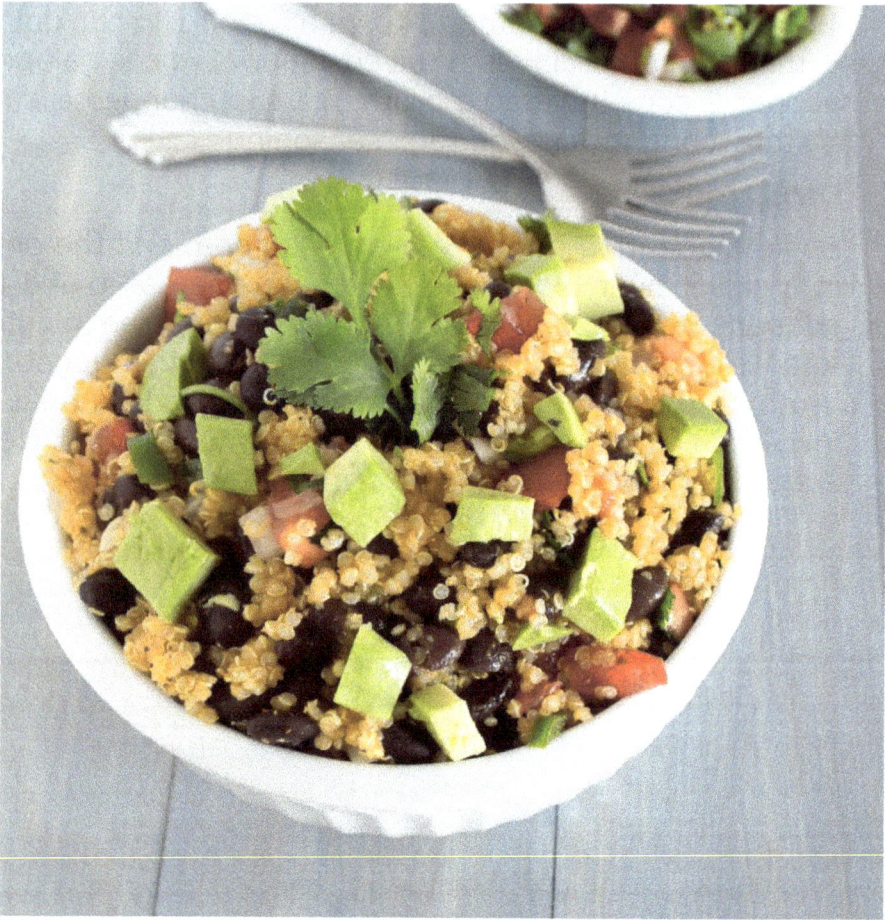

Pesky Pesto Quinoa

Preparation time: 10 minutes Cooking time: 40 minutesServings: 4.

Ingredients:

1 ¼ cup quinoa 2 diced tomatoes 3 cups vegetable broth 3 tbsp. basil pesto

Directions:

Begin by allowing the quinoa and the broth to boil in a saucepan. Next, cover the saucepan, and simmer the ingredients for twenty minutes. Remove the saucepan from the heat and add the quinoa and the tomato. Add salt and pepper as you please, and serve warm. Enjoy.

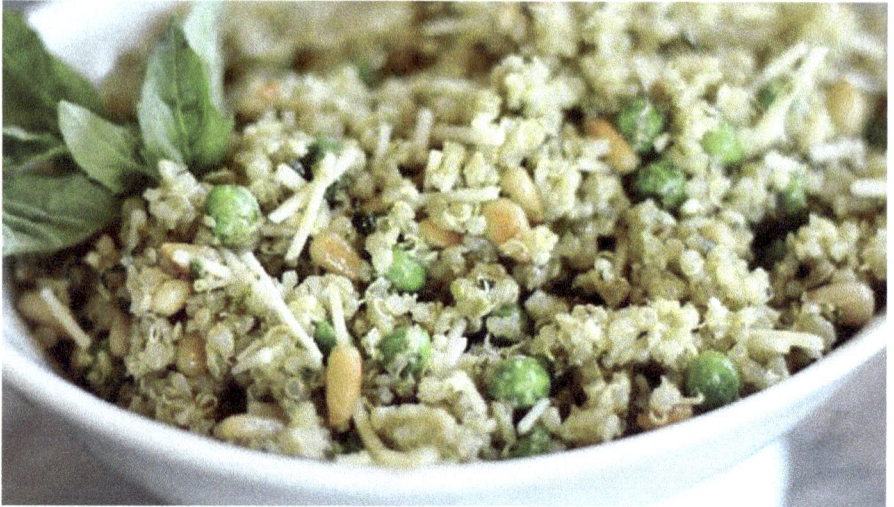

Chived Vegan Sour Cream Mashed Potatoes

Preparation time: 10 minutes Cooking time: 20 minutesServings: 8.

Ingredients:

3 pounds quartered Yukon gold potatoes ½ cup soymilk ¾ cup vegan sour cream 1/3 cup minced chives salt and pepper to taste

Directions:

Begin by placing the potatoes in a pot with water. Allow the potatoes to simmer for thirty minutes. Next, drain the pot and mash the potatoes with the rest of the ingredients. Utilize a masher or a mixer to get your desired consistency. Season the potatoes with salt and pepper, and enjoy.

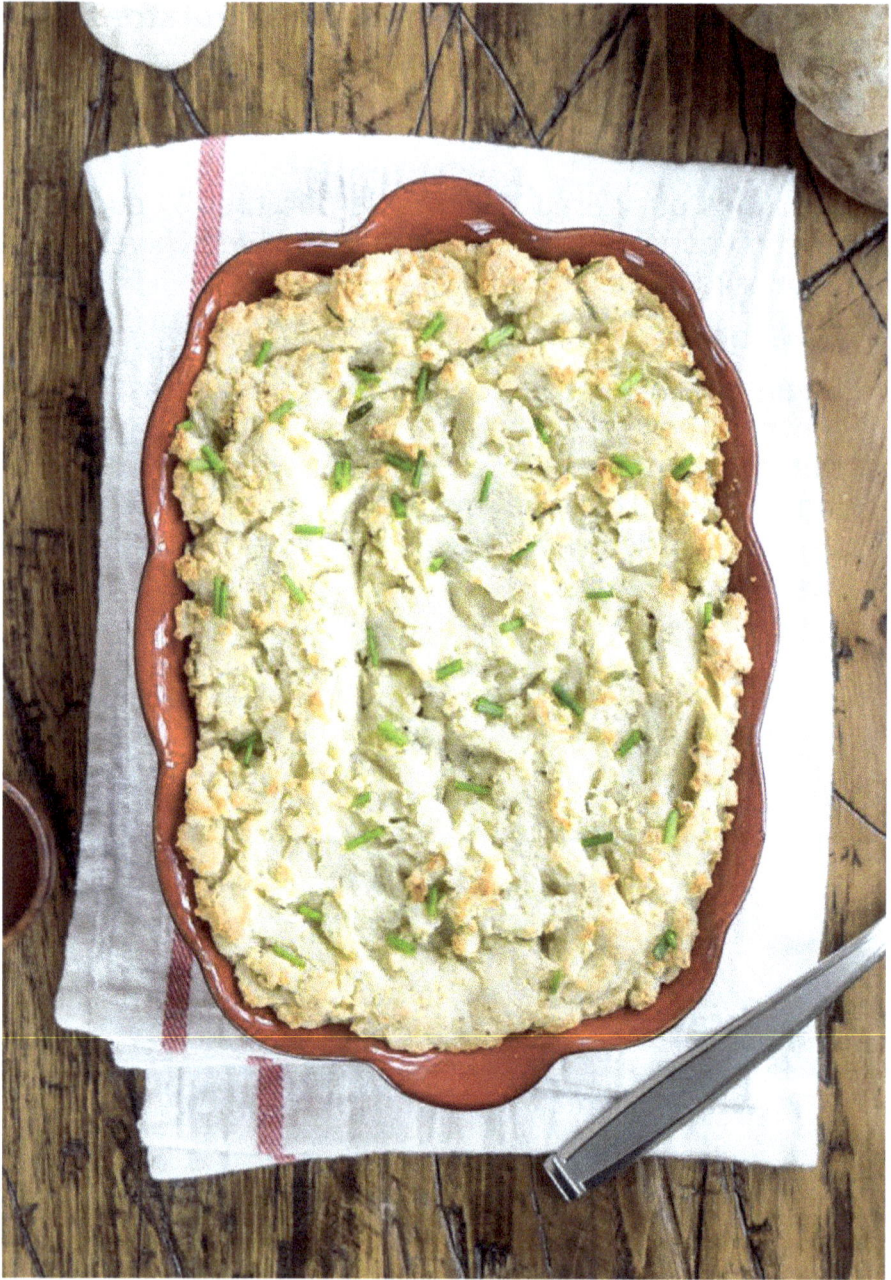

Cheezin' Potato Faux Pancakes

Preparation time: 10 minutes Cooking time: 50 minutesServings: 6.

Ingredients:

5 grated potatoes 3 egg replacements ½ cup soymilk 1 tsp. onion powder ½ cup grated vegan Parmesan cheese 1 cup flour ½ cup grated vegan cheddar cheese 1 tsp. baking powder 1/3 cup corn oil 2 tbsp. vegan butter salt and pepper to taste

Directions:

Begin by mixing together the potatoes, the egg replacements, and the soymilk in a big mixing bowl. Add the vegan cheese, the flour, the onion powder, the baking powder, the salt, and the pepper. Stir well and assimilate with a fork. Next, place the corn oil and the vegan butter together in a skillet, and heat the mixture well. Add 3 tbsp. of potato mixture to the skillet to make patties. Cook the patties for five minutes on each side, and drain them on paper towels before serving. Enjoy.

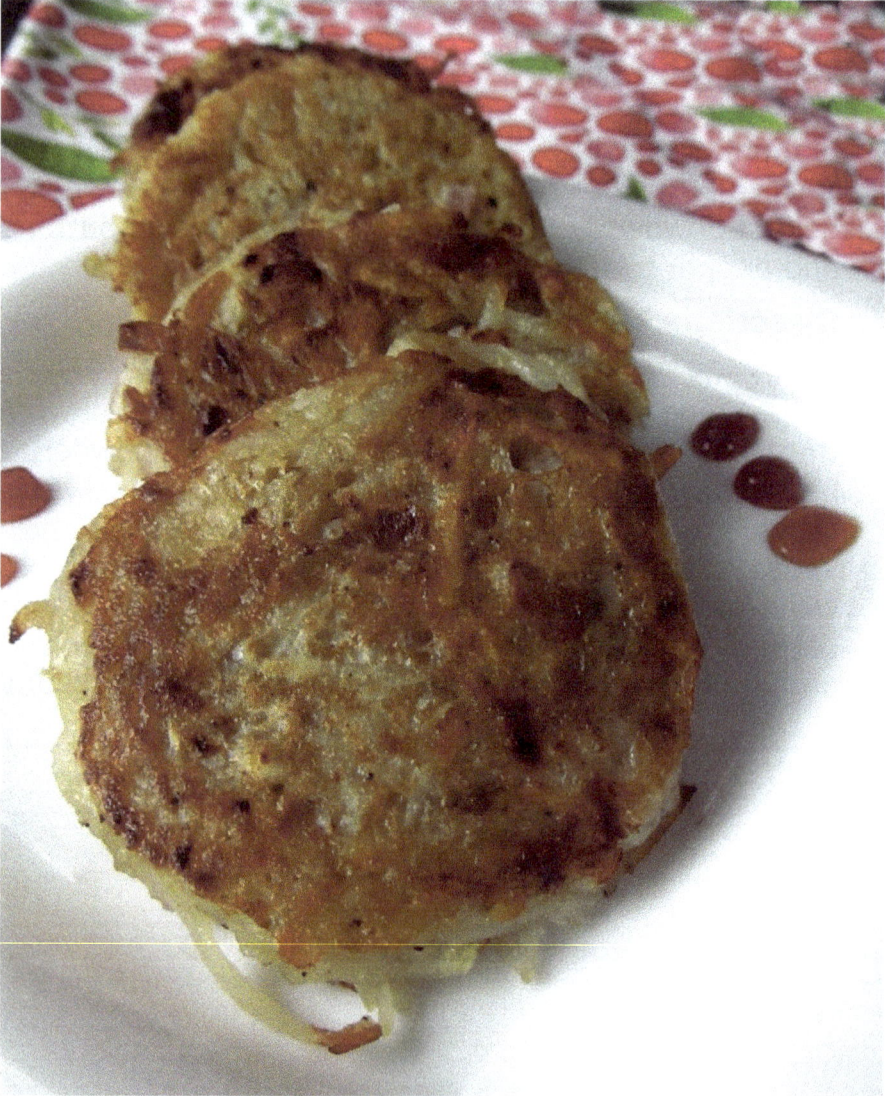

Cashewed Rice Pilaf

Preparation time: 10 minutes Cooking time: 35 minutesServings: 12.

Ingredients:

1 cup wild rice 1/3 cup vegan butter 2 cups long grain rice 3 cups frozen peas 1 diced onion 4 ounces died pimento peppers 2 diced carrots 1 ½ cup golden raisins 1 cup cashews 4 cups vegetable broth salt and pepper to taste

Direction:

Begin by placing the butter in a saucepan and melting it over medium. Add the long rice, the carrot, the raisins, and the onion together for five minutes. Next, add the broth and allow the mixture to boil. Then, cover the mixture and allow it to simmer on low for twenty-five minutes. To the side, allow 2 cups of water to boil. Add the wild rice and allow it to simmer for forty-five minutes. Next, add the wild rice, the pimentos, the peas, and the cashews to the raisined mixture, and heat on the stovetop at medium. Serve warm, and enjoy.

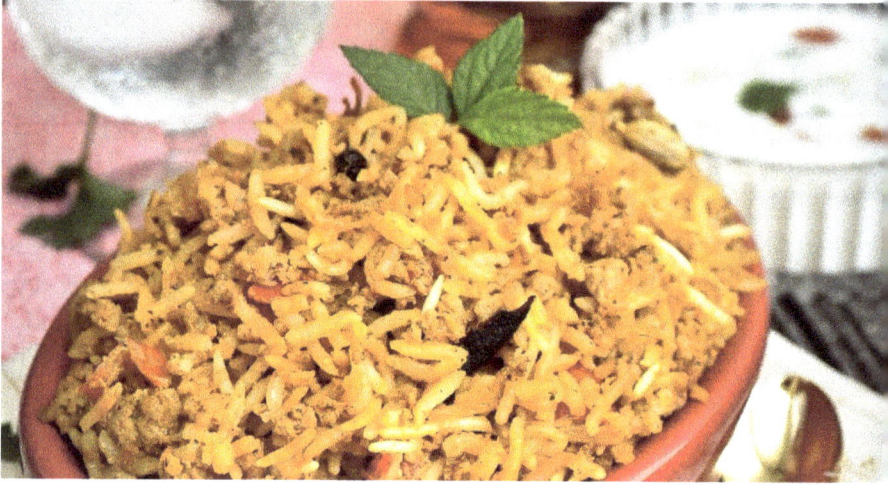

Mediterranean Garbanzo-Bean Fritters

Preparation time: 10 minutes Cooking time: 25 minutes Servings: 4.

Ingredients:

1 cup garbanzo bean flour 1 tsp. salt ½ tsp. cumin 1 ¼ cup chopped spinach ¼ tsp. baking soda 4 minced garlic cloves 2 sliced scallions 1 cup drained garbanzo beans 1 cup olive oil

Directions: Begin by preheating the oven to 200 degrees Fahrenheit. Next, stir together the flour, salt, and cumin. Add hot water a little bit at a time in order to create a paste-like texture: like pancake batter. Allow this mixture to stand at room temperature for one hour. Afterwards, add the baking soda, the garlic, and the spinach to the mixture. Stir. Next, add the scallions and the chickpeas. Pour the olive oil in the skillet, and place the heat on medium. When you've heated the oil sufficiently, place the fritters on the oil and brown them for three minutes on each side. Drain the fritters on paper towels, and serve them with your favorite dipping sauce.

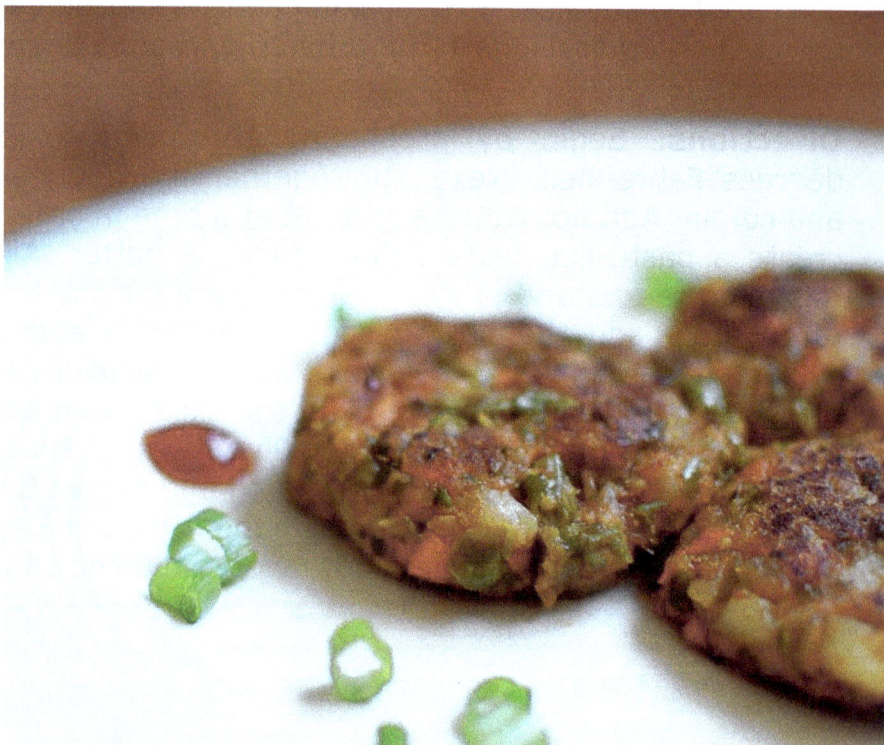

Asian-Inspired Summer Goi Cuan

Preparation time: 10 minutes Cooking time: 30 minutes 24 rolls.

Ingredients:

24 round rice paper wrappers 6-7 cups of jasmine tea 2 de-ribbed and separated lettuce heads 9 ounces cooked thin rice vermicelli noodles ½ cup Thai basil leaves 1 ½ cups enoki mushrooms 1 cup chopped mint ¼ cup chopped cilantro ½ cup sliced scallions 2 sliced carrots 1 sliced cucumber

Directions:

Begin by preparing the tea and keeping it warm. Next, dip each of the rice paper wrappers into the tea. Place the rice wrappers on a cutting board, and place a layer of lettuce in the center. Enter in a bit of all of the above ingredients. Next, fold over the bottom of the rice paper overtop of the filling. Tuck in the sides, and continue to wrap the rice up. Do this for each of the 24 rice paper wrappers, and chill the rolls prior to serving. Enjoy!

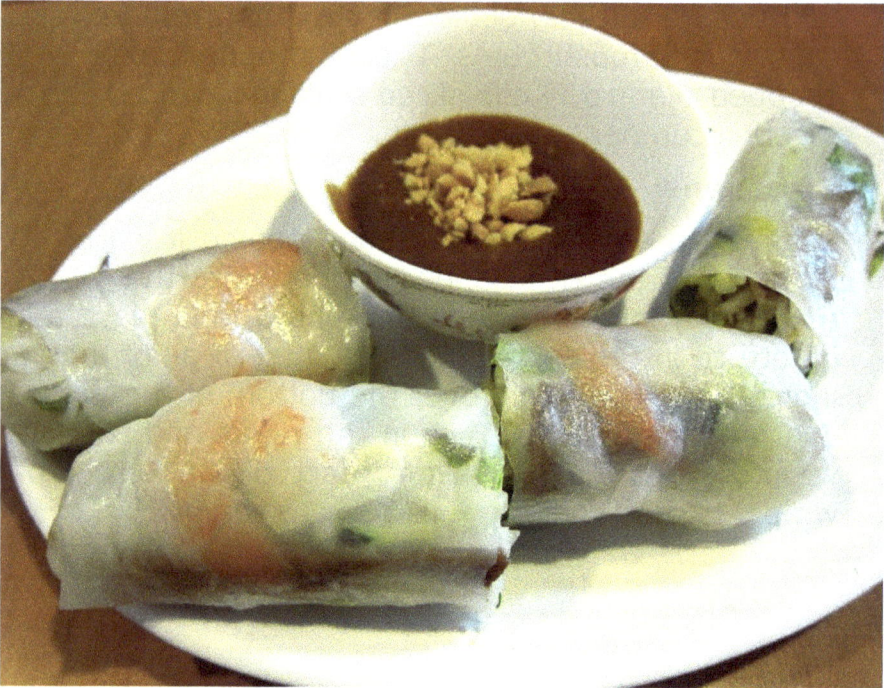

Yummy Roasted Mushrooms

Preparation time: 10 minutes Cooking time: 30 minutes 8 Servings.

Ingredients:

2 pounds cremini mushrooms 2 ½ tbsp. olive oil 2 tbsp. soy sauce 2 minced garlic cloves spinach for serving

Directions:

Begin by preheating the oven to 350 degrees Fahrenheit. Slice up the mushrooms, and place the mushrooms in a large mixing bowl with the rest of the ingredients—except for the spinach. Bake the ingredients in a baking dish for thirty minutes. Next, remove the baked ingredients, and place them overtop of the spinach in a serving bowl. Enjoy.

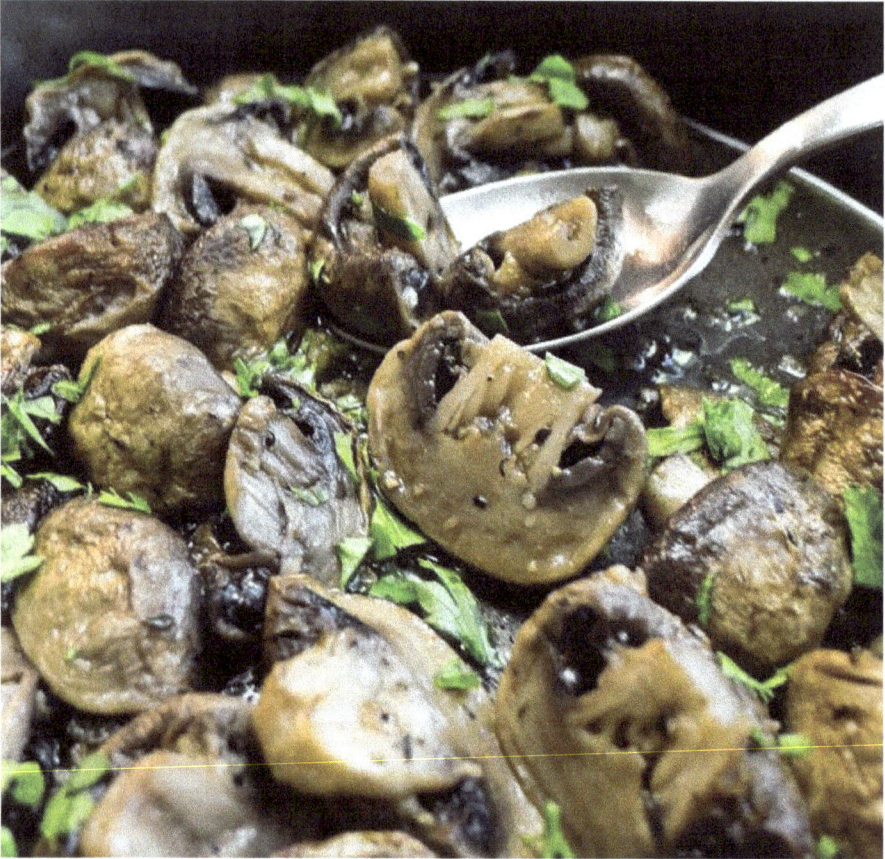

Savory Scallion Pancakes

Preparation time: 10 minutes Cooking time: 20 minutes 24 mini pancakes.

Ingredients:

1 cup spelt flour 1 cup and 2 tbsp. rice milk 1 cup sliced scallions 1 tsp. salt olive oil for cooking

Directions:

Begin by combining the above ingredients in a mixing bowl. Stir the ingredients well until they're smooth. Afterwards, oil up a griddle and place about 1/8 of a cup of batter on the griddle for each pancake. Cook each side of the pancake to achieve a golden brown color. Next, place the pancakes on a plate, and cover the pancakes while you continue to cook the rest of the batter. Place the pancakes out on a nice platter, and serve warm.

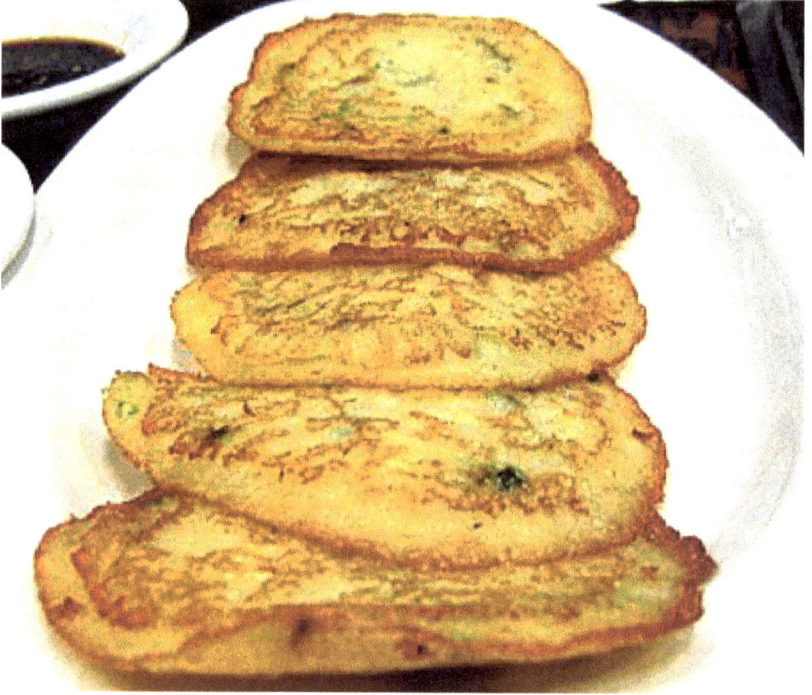

Smokin' Peanut and Tofu

Preparation time: 10 minutes Cooking time: 60 minutes 10 servings.

Ingredients:

7 ounces smoked tofu 6 celery stalks 2 ounces roasted peanuts 3 tbsp. chili oil ½ tsp. sugar salt to taste

Directions:

Begin by slicing the tofu into small cubes and squeezing them of their water. Afterwards, slice up the celery into small strips the same size as the small tofu squares. Allow water to boil in a small saucepan. Add the celery and allow it to blanch for one minute. Afterwards, remove the celery and allow it to cool. Shake it dry. Bring all the above ingredients together in a bowl for an essential appetizer. Enjoy!

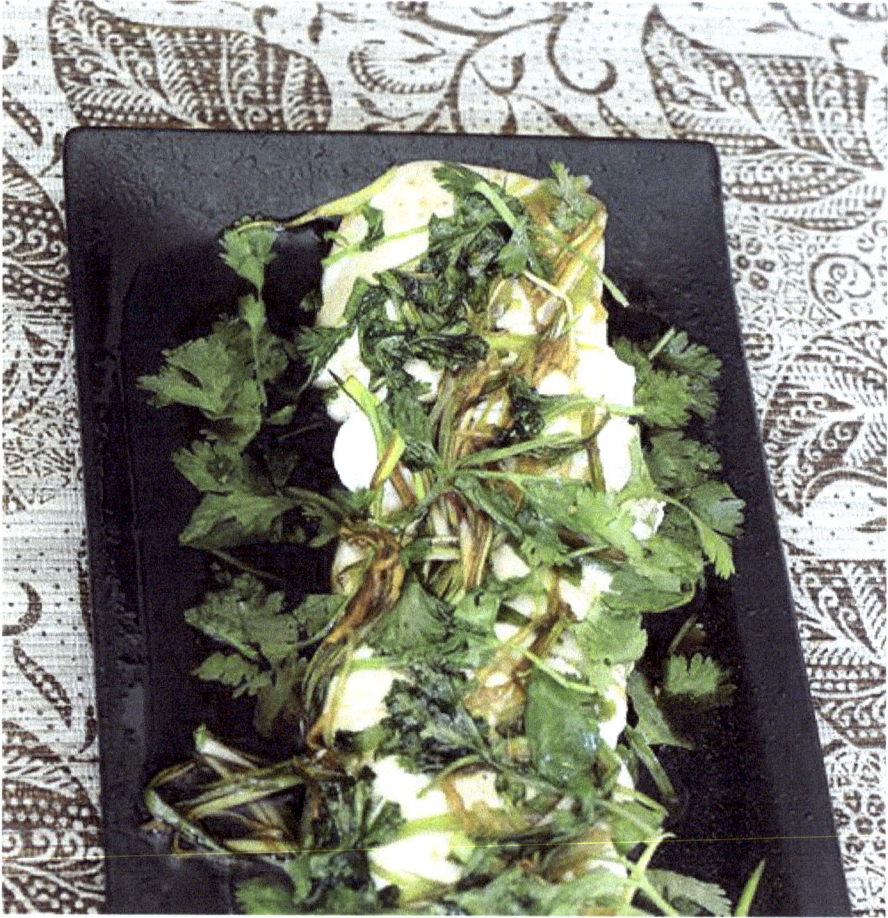

Artichoke Attack Appetizer

Preparation time: 10 minutes Cooking time: 40 minutes 6 Servings.

Ingredients:

10 ounces asparagus 8 ounces button mushrooms 8 ounces artichoke hearts 1 chopped dill pickle 1 sliced zucchini ¼ cup chopped parsley ½ cup vegan mayonnaise (recipe here) 1 juiced lemon salt and pepper to taste

Directions:

Begin by slicing up the mushrooms and placing them in a skillet with about ¼ cup water. Cover the skillet and allow them to steam on medium-heat for two and a half minutes. Next, drain the mushrooms and allow them to cool. To the side, trim at the bottom of the asparagus, and slice the asparagus into smaller, one-inch pieces. Place the asparagus in the mushroom skillet, and place just about three tbsp.. of water at the bottom. Steam the asparagus until the asparagus is a bright green. Drain the asparagus, and rinse it. Bring the mushrooms and asparagus together in a serving bowl. Bring in the artichoke hearts, the dill pickle, the zucchini, the parsley, the mayonnaise, the lemon, and the salt and pepper, Mix well, and enjoy.

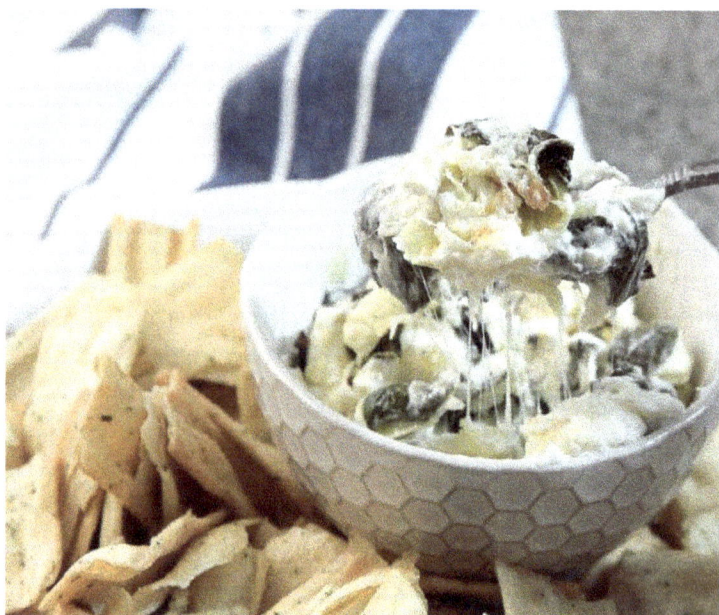

Lucky Lemon Mushrooms

Preparation time: 10 minutes Cooking time: 20 minutes 6 Servings.

Ingredients:

1 tsp. agave nectar 3 tbsp. lemon juice 1 tbsp. olive oil 2 minced garlic cloves 10 ounces sliced portabella mushrooms

Directions:

Bring together the agave nectar, the lemon juice, the olive oil, and the minced garlic in a mixing bowl. Place the sliced mushrooms in the created mixture, and stir them together. Next, place the mushrooms in a baking pan, and pour the marinade overtop of them. Broil the mushrooms for four minutes. After four minutes, stir the mushrooms. Broil them for an additional five minutes. The mushrooms should be darker. Remove the mushrooms, and serve them warm. Enjoy!

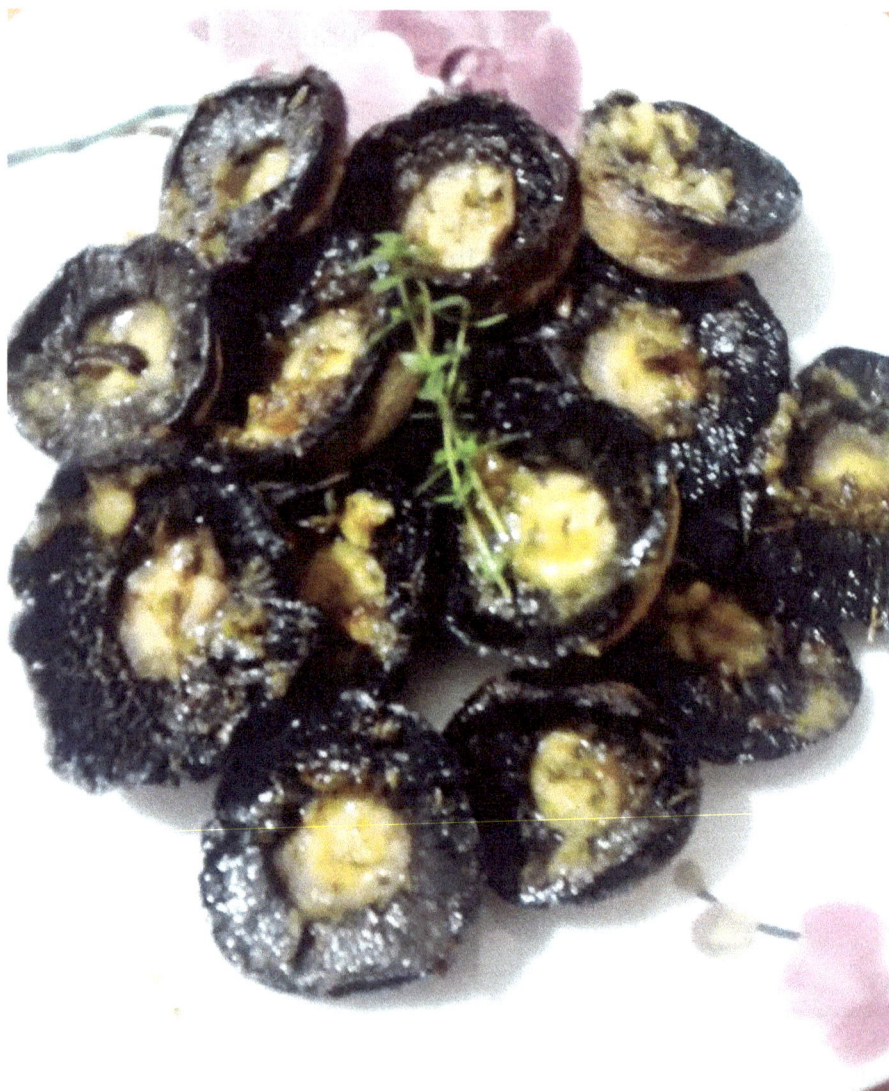

Pesto Stuffed Mushrooms

Preparation time: 20 minutes Cooking time: 25 minutes Servings: 6

Ingredients:

6 large cremini mushrooms 6 bacon slices 2 tablespoons basil pesto 5 tablespoons low-fat cream cheese softened What you'll need from the store cupboard: None

Directions:

Line a cookie sheet with foil and preheat oven to 375oF. In a small bowl mix well, pesto and cream cheese. Remove stems of mushrooms and discard. Evenly fill mushroom caps with pesto-cream cheese filling. Get one stuffed mushroom and a slice of bacon. Wrap the bacon all over the mushrooms. Repeat process on remaining mushrooms and bacon. Place bacon-wrapped mushrooms on prepared pan and bake for 25 minutes or until bacon is crispy. Let it cool, evenly divide into suggested servings, and enjoy.

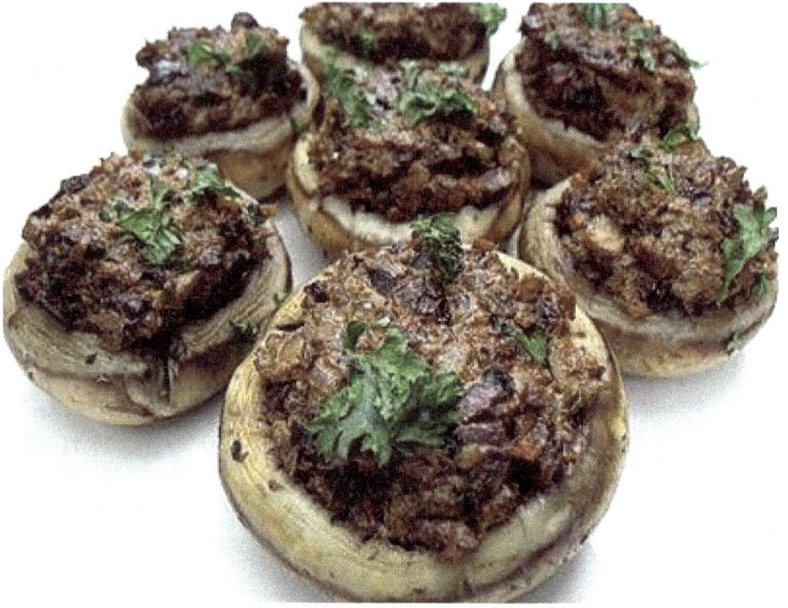

Delicious Potato Mix

Preparation Time: 10 minutes Cooking Time: 25 minutes Servings:

Ingredients

6 ounces jarred roasted red bell peppers, chopped 3 garlic cloves, minced 2 tablespoons parsley, chopped Salt and black pepper to the taste 2 tablespoons chives, chopped 4 potatoes, peeled and cut into wedges Cooking spray

Directions:

In a pan that fits your Air Fryer, combine roasted bell peppers with garlic, parsley, salt, pepper, chives, potato wedges and the oil, toss, transfer to your Air Fryer and cook at 350 °F for 25 minutes. Divide between plates and serve as a side dish.

Easy Portobello Mushrooms

Preparation Time: 10 minutes Cooking Time: 12 minutes Servings:

Ingredients

4 big Portobello mushroom caps 1 tablespoon olive oil 1 cup spinach, torn 1/3 cup vegan breadcrumbs ¼ teaspoon rosemary, chopped

Directions:

Rub mushrooms caps with the oil, place them in your Air Fryer's basket and cook them at 350 ° F for 2 minutes. Meanwhile, in a bowl, mix spinach, rosemary and breadcrumbs and stir well. Stuff mushrooms with this mix, place them in your Air Fryer's basket again and cook at 350 ° F for 10 minutes. Divide them between plates and serve as a side dish.

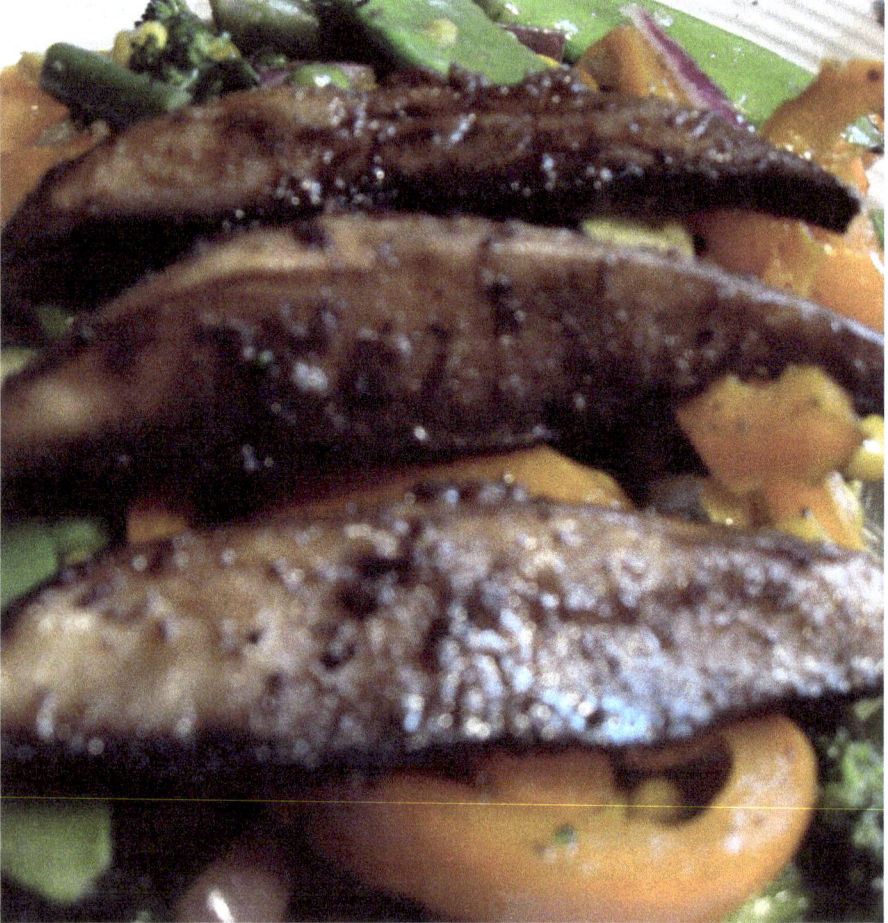

Sweet Potatoes Side Dish

Preparation Time: 10 minutes Cooking time: 3 hours Servings: 10

Ingredients:

4 pounds sweet potatoes, thinly sliced 3 tablespoons stevia ½ cup orange juice ½ teaspoon sage, dried 2 tablespoons olive oil

Directions:

Arrange potato slices on the bottom of your slow cooker. Add this over potatoes, cover slow cooker and cook on High for 3 hours. Divide between

plates and serve as a side dish. Enjoy!

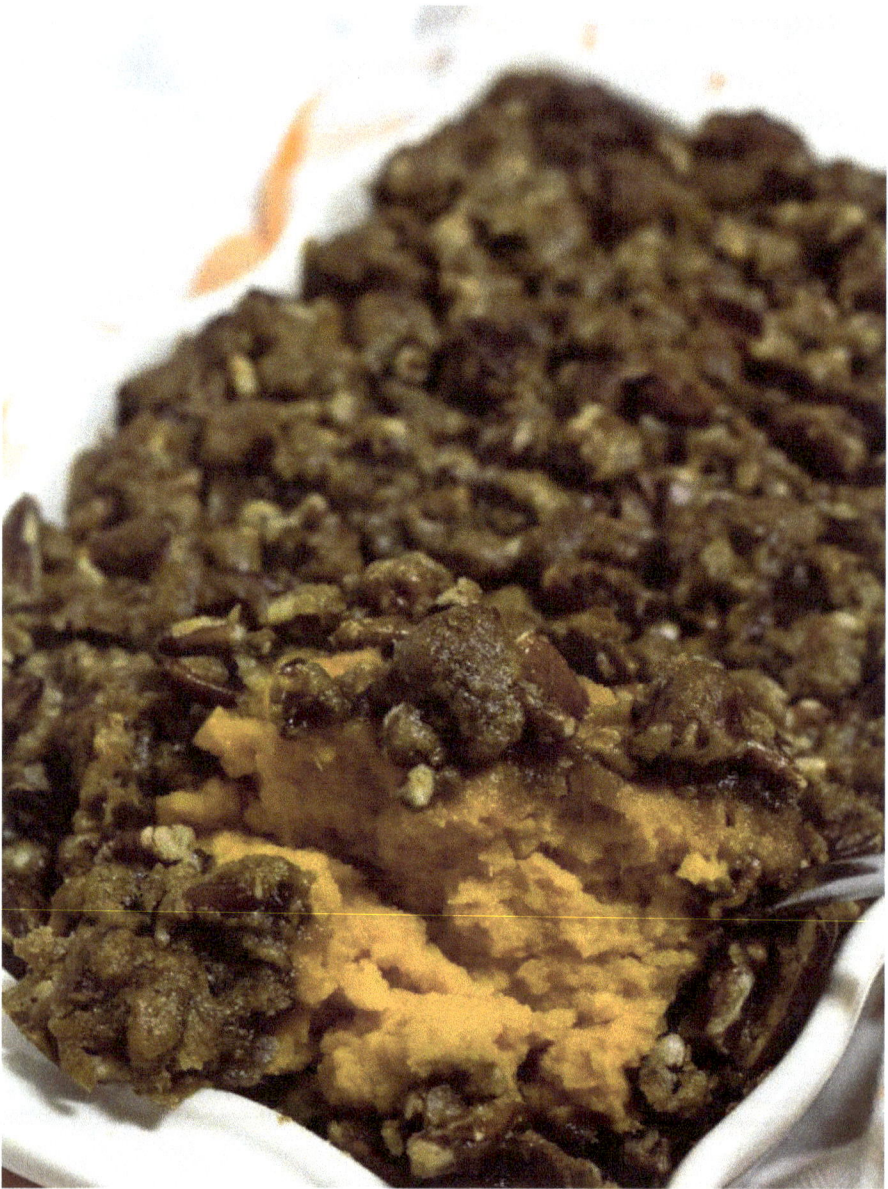

Wild Rice Mix

Preparation Time: 10 minutes Cooking time: 6 hours Servings: 12

Ingredients:

40 ounces veggie stock 2 and ½ cups wild rice 1 cup carrot, shredded 4 ounces mushrooms, sliced 2 tablespoons olive oil 2 teaspoons marjoram, dried and crushed Salt and black pepper to the taste 2/3 cup dried cherries ½ cup pecans, toasted and chopped 2/3 cup green onions, chopped

Directions:

In your slow cooker, mix stock with wild rice, carrot, mushrooms, oil, marjoram, salt, pepper, cherries, pecans and green onions, toss, cover and cook on Low for 6 hours. Stir wild rice one more time, divide between plates and serve as a side dish. Enjoy!

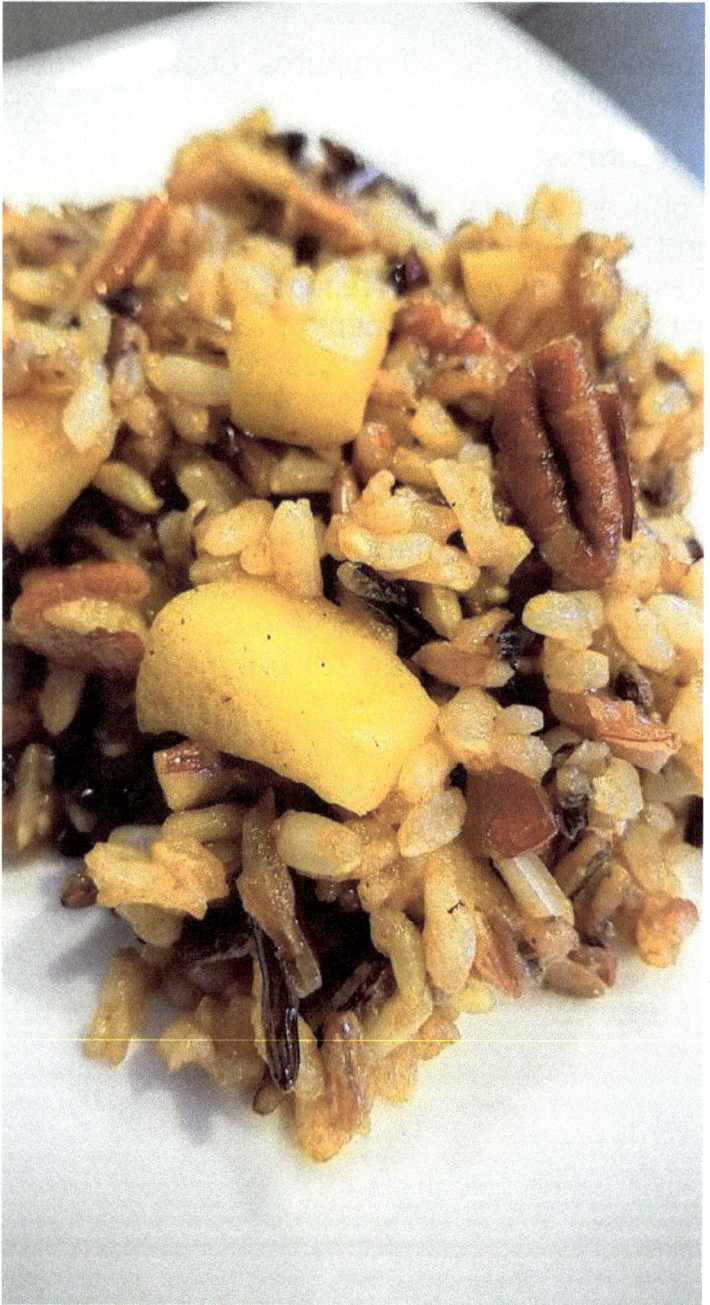

Thai Peanut Zucchini Noodle Salad

Preparation Time: 10 minutes Cooking Time: 10 minutes
Serving Yields: 4

Ingredients:

Medium zucchini - 3 spiralized Carrot – 1 spiralized
Chopped green onions - .25 cup Extra firm tofu, drained
and cubed - .5 of 1 block Skinny Peanut Sauce 5 cup +1-
2 tbsp.water Peanuts 5 cup

Ingredients for the sauce:

Protein Plus peanut flour - .25 cup Ginger – 1 tsp. Garlic
powder - .5 tsp. Low-sodium soy sauce - gluten-free, if
desired – 2 tbsp. Lakanto Liquid Monkfruit Sweetener or
another liquid sweetener - 6 drops or to taste Lime juice
- juice of 2 limes - 1 tbsp. Water - add more if desired –
2 tbsp. Ingredients for the salad: Spiralized carrot- 1
Medium spiralized zucchini - 3 Diced green onions - .25
cup Extra-firm tofu - .5 of a block Skinny Peanut Sauce-
.5 cup plus 1-2 Tbsp water Peanuts - .5 cup

Directions:

Drain and cube the tofu. Prepare the sauce by adding the
water until it's like you like it. Combine the remainder of
the fixings except for the peanuts in another container.
Top it off with the prepared salad dressing, and toss well.
Sprinkle using some of the peanuts, and serve.

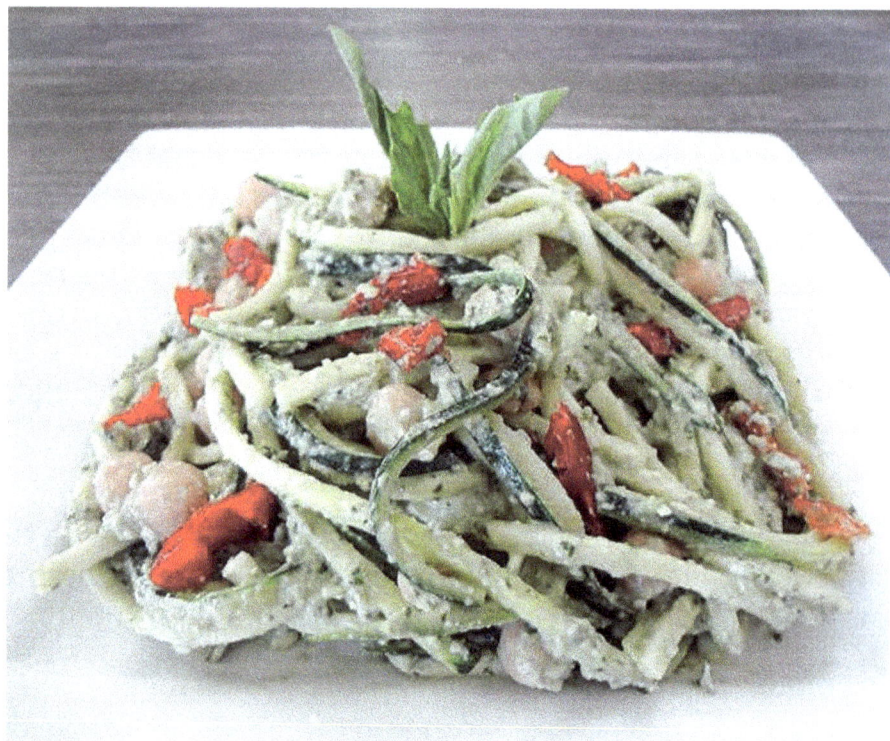

Almond Butter Brownies

Preparation Time: 30 minutes Serves: 4

Ingredients:

1 scoop protein powder 2 tbsp cocoa powder 1/2 cup almond butter, melted 1 cup bananas, overripe

Directions:

Preheat the oven to 350 F/ 176 C. Spray brownie tray with cooking spray. Add all Ingredients into the blender and blend until smooth. Pour batter into the prepared dish and bake in preheated oven for 20 minutes. Serve and enjoy.

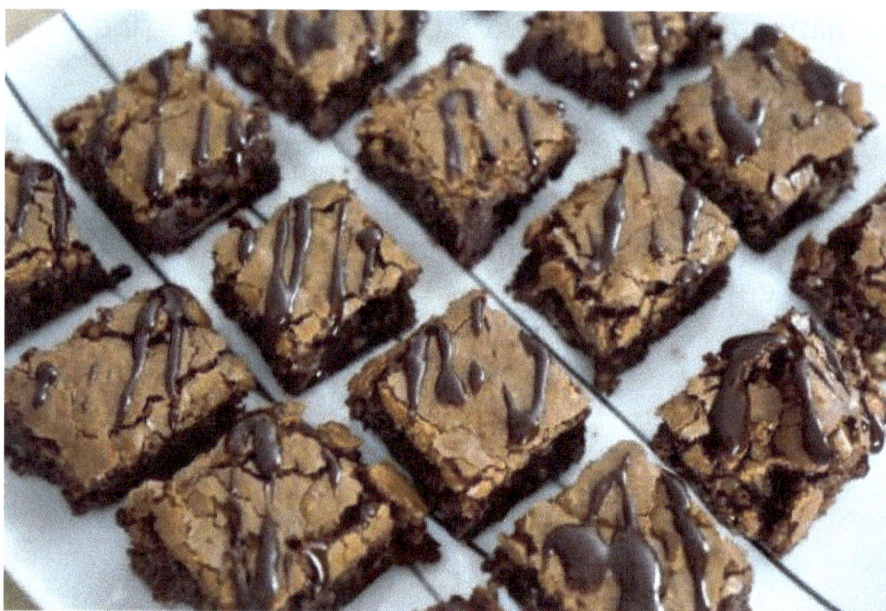

Quick Chocó Brownie

Preparation Time: 10 minutes Serves: 1 Ingredients: 1/4 cup almond milk 1 tbsp cocoa powder 1 scoop chocolate protein powder 1/2 tsp baking powder

Directions:

In a microwave-safe mug blend together baking powder, protein powder, and cocoa. Add almond milk in a mug and stir well. Place mug in microwave and microwave for 30 seconds. Serve and enjoy.

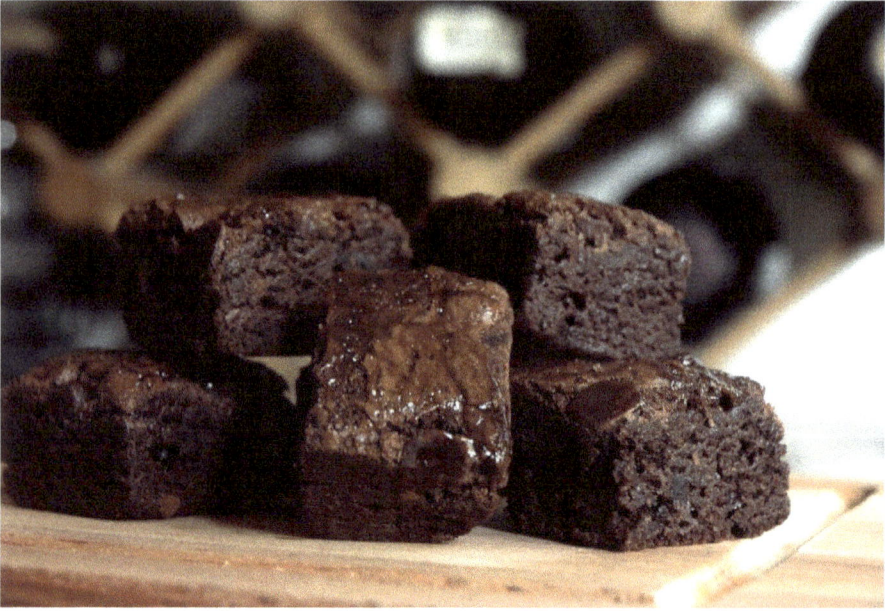

Coconut Peanut Butter Fudge

Preparation Time: 1 hour 15 minutes Serves: 20

Ingredients:

12 oz smooth peanut butter 3 tbsp coconut oil 4 tbsp coconut cream 15 drops liquid stevia Pinch of salt

Directions:

Line baking tray with parchment paper. Melt coconut oil in a saucepan over low heat. Add peanut butter, coconut cream, stevia, and salt in a saucepan. Stir well. Pour fudge mixture into the prepared baking tray and place in refrigerator for 1 hour. Cut into pieces and serve.

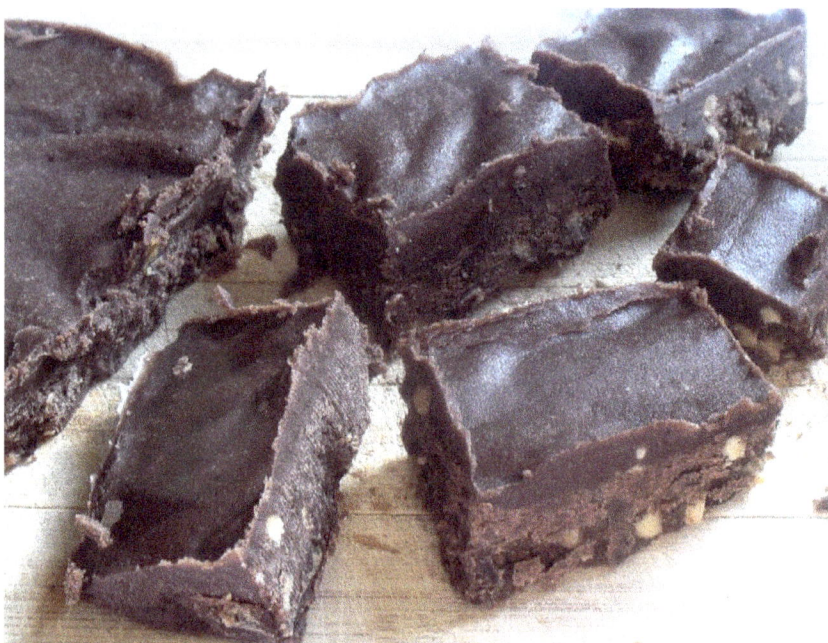

Chocó Chia Pudding

Preparation Time: 10 minutes Serves: 6

Ingredients:

2 1/2 cups coconut milk 2 scoops stevia extract powder 6 tbsp cocoa powder 1/2 cup chia seeds 1/2 tsp vanilla extract 1/8 cup xylitol 1/8 tsp salt

Directions: Add all Ingredients into the blender and blend until smooth. Pour mixture into the glass container and place in refrigerator. Serve chilled and enjoy.

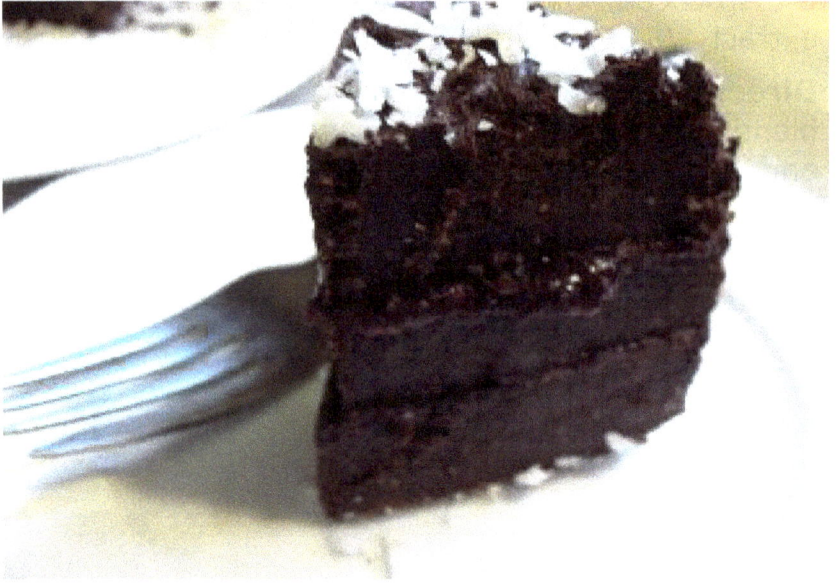

Carrot and Radish Slaw with Sesame Dressing

Preparation Time: 10 minutes Cooking Time: 0 minute Servings: 4

Ingredients:

2 tablespoons sesame oil, toasted 3 tablespoons rice vinegar ½ teaspoon sugar 2 tablespoons low sodium tamari 1 cup carrots, sliced into strips 2 cups radishes, sliced 2 tablespoons fresh cilantro, chopped 2 teaspoons sesame seeds, toasted

Direction

Mix the oil, vinegar, sugar and tamari in a bowl. Add the carrots, radishes and cilantro. Toss to coat evenly. Let sit for 10 minutes. Transfer to a food container.

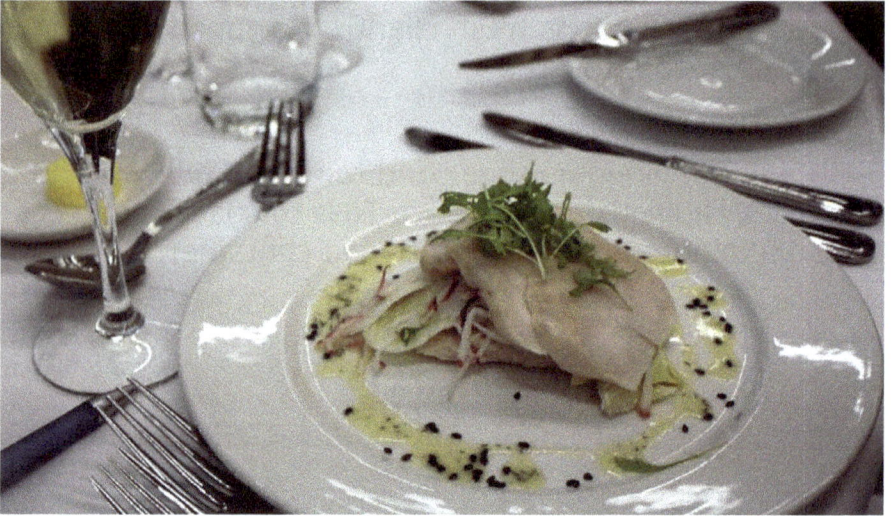

Roasted Veggies in Lemon Sauce

Preparation Time: 15 minutes Cooking Time: 20 minutes Servings: 5

Ingredients:

2 cloves garlic, sliced 1 ½ cups broccoli florets 1 ½ cups cauliflower florets 1 tablespoon olive oil Salt to taste 1 teaspoon dried oregano, crushed ¾ cup zucchini, diced ¾ cup red bell pepper, diced 2 teaspoons lemon zest

Direction

Preheat your oven to 425 degrees F. In a baking pan, add the garlic, broccoli and cauliflower. Toss in oil and season with salt and oregano. Roast in the oven for 10 minutes. Add the zucchini and bell pepper to the pan. Stir well. Roast for another 10 minutes. Sprinkle lemon zest on top before serving. Transfer to a food container and reheat before serving.

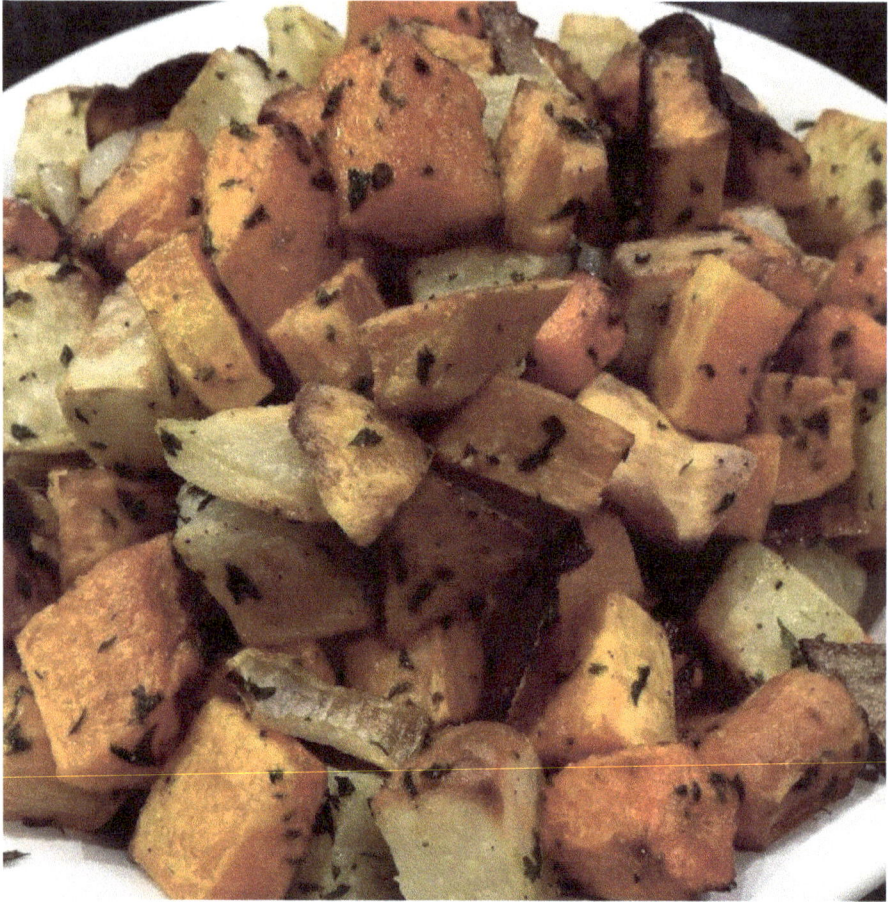

Vegan Tacos

Preparation Time: 20 minutes Cooking Time: 10 minutes
Servings: 4

Ingredients:

½ teaspoon onion powder ½ teaspoon garlic powder 1 teaspoon chili powder 2 tablespoons tamari 16 oz. tofu, drained and crumbled 1 tablespoon olive oil 1 ripe avocado 1 tablespoon vegan mayonnaise 1 teaspoon lime juice Salt to taste 8 corn tortillas, warmed ½ cup fresh salsa 2 cups iceberg lettuce, shredded Pickled radishes

Direction

Combine the onion powder, garlic powder, chili powder and tamari in a bowl. Marinate the tofu in the mixture for 10 minutes. Pour the oil in a pan over medium heat. Cook the tofu mixture for 10 minutes. In another bowl, mash the avocado and mix with mayo, lime juice and salt. Stuff each corn tortilla with tofu mixture, mashed avocado, salsa and lettuce. Serve with pickled radishes.

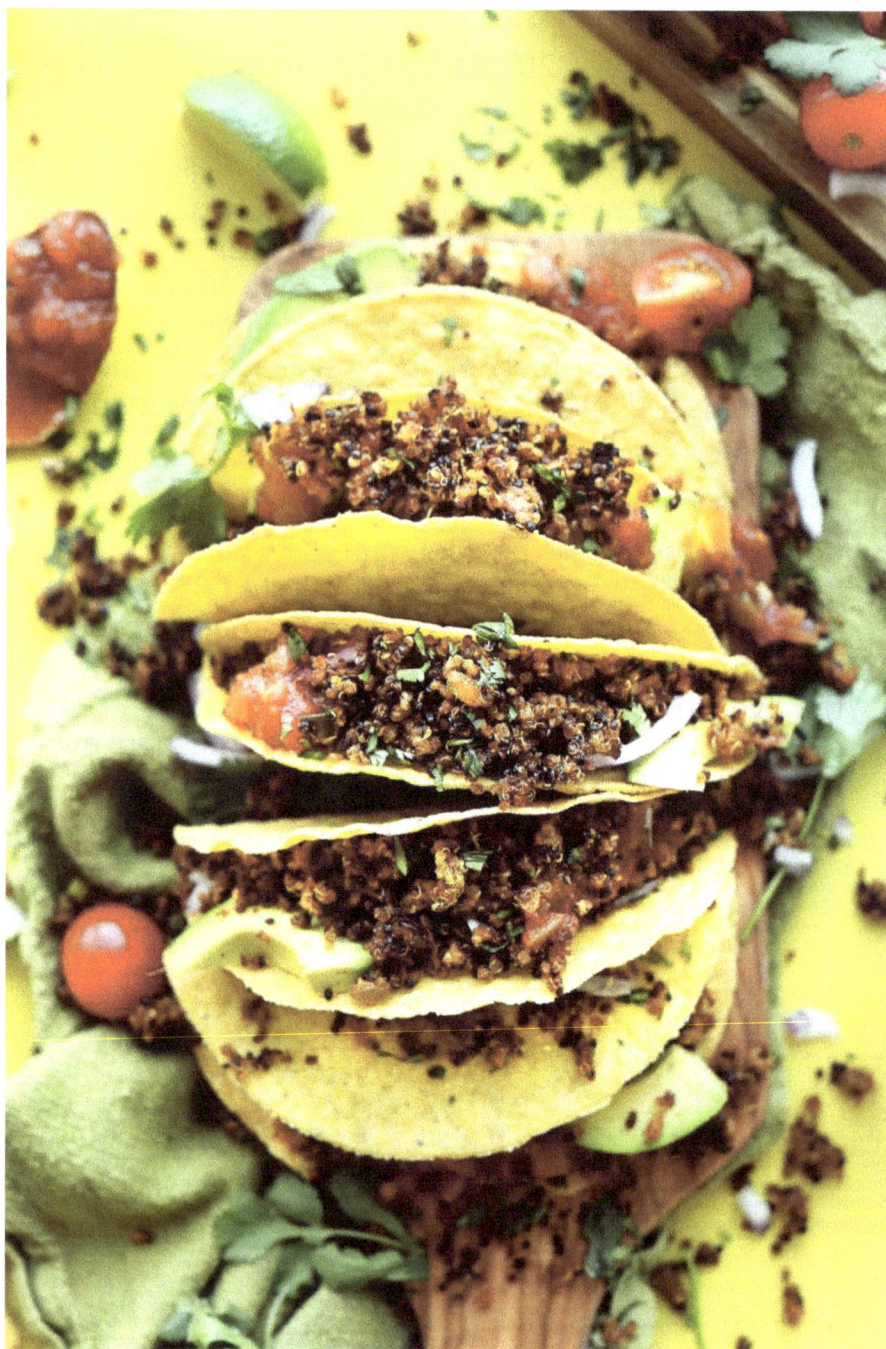

Tomato Basil Pasta

Preparation Time: 5 minutes Cooking Time: 10 minutes Servings: 4

Ingredients:

2 cups low-sodium vegetable broth 2 cups water 8 oz. pasta 1 ½ teaspoons Italian seasoning 15 oz. canned diced tomatoes 2 tablespoons olive oil ½ teaspoon garlic powder ½ teaspoon onion powder ¼ teaspoon crushed red pepper ½ teaspoon salt 6 cups baby spinach ½ cup basil, chopped

Direction

Add all the Ingredients except spinach and basil in a pot over high heat. Mix well. Cover the pot and bring to a boil. Reduce the heat. Simmer for 5 minutes. Add the spinach and cook for 5 more minutes. Stir in basil. Transfer to a food container. Microwave before serving.

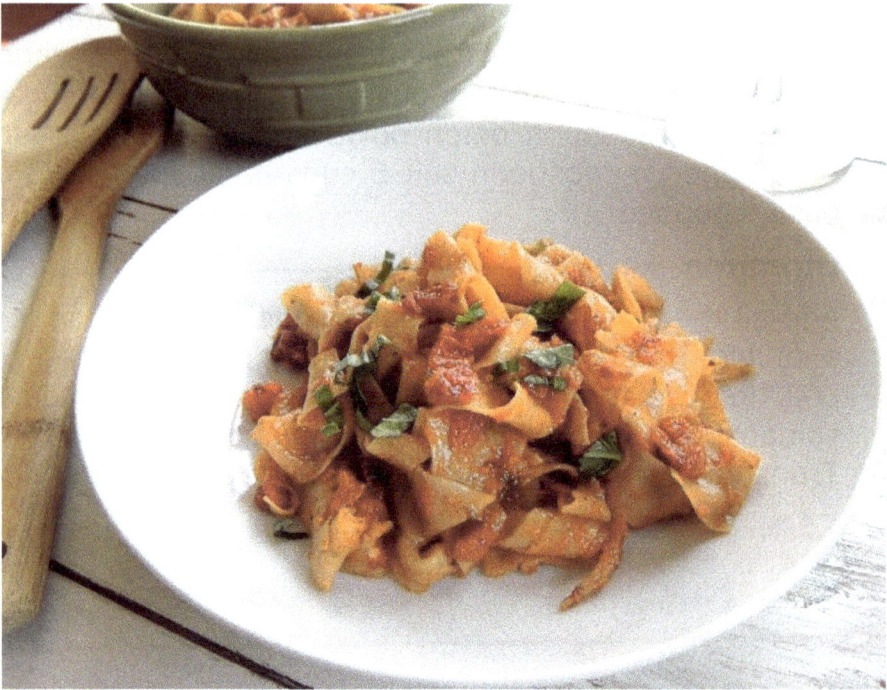

Tofu Shawarma Rice

Preparation Time: 15 minutes Cooking Time: 15 minutes Servings: 4

Ingredients:

4 cups cooked brown rice 4 cups cooked tofu, sliced into small cubes 4 cups cucumber, cubed 4 cups tomatoes, cubed 4 cups white onion, cubed 2 cups cabbage, shredded 1/2 cup vegan mayo 1/8 cup garlic, minced Garlic salt to taste Hot sauce

Direction

Add brown rice into 4 food containers. Arrange tofu, cucumber, tomatoes, white onion and cabbage on top. In a bowl, mix the mayo, garlic, and garlic salt. Drizzle top with garlic sauce and hot sauce before serving.

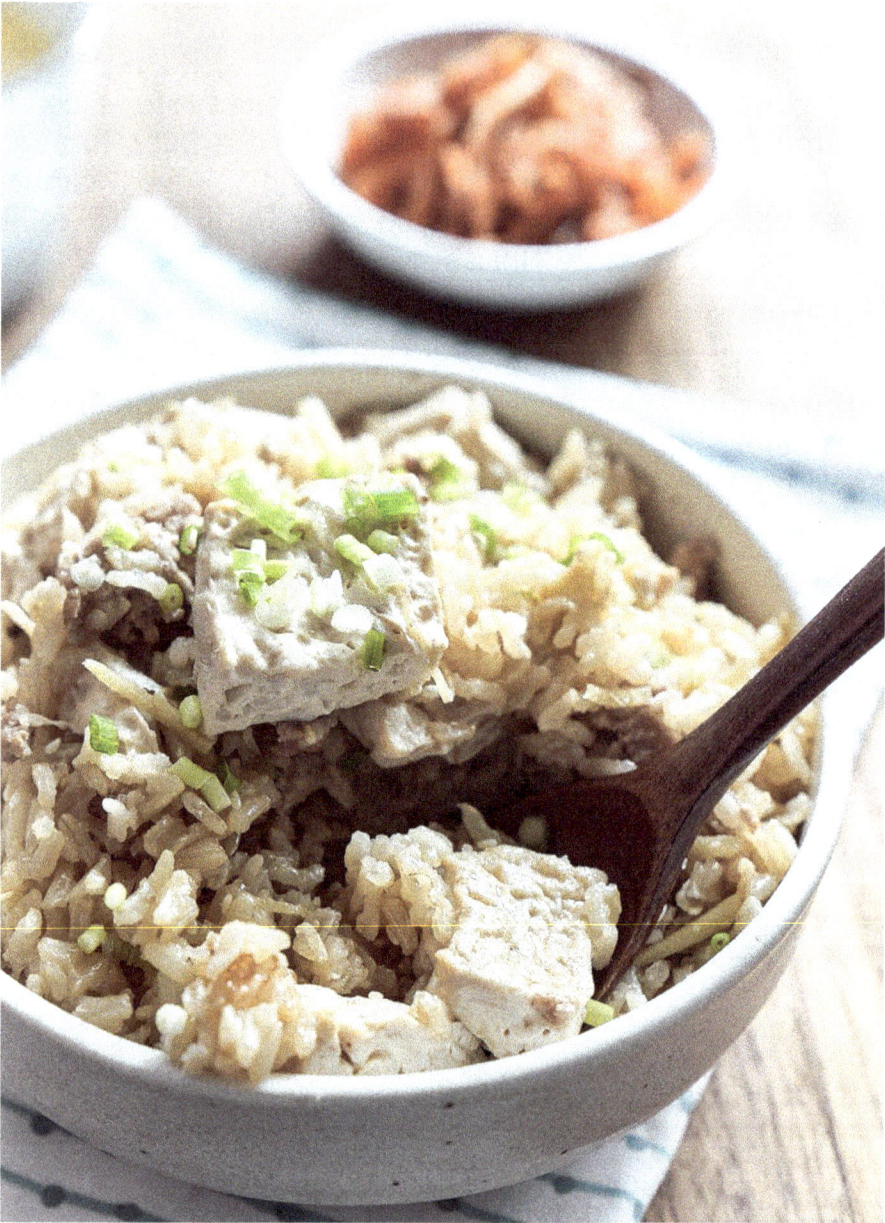

Cheesy" Spinach Rolls

Preparation Time: 20 minutes Cooking Time: 15 minutes Servings: 6

Ingredients:

18 spinach leaves 18 vegan spring roll wrappers 6 slices cheese, cut into 18 smaller strips Water 1 cup vegetable oil 6 cups cauliflower rice 3 cups tomato, cubed 3 cups cucumber, cubed 1 tablespoon olive oil 1 teaspoon balsamic vinegar

Direction

Place one spinach leaf on top of each wrapper. Add a small strip of vegan cheese on top of each spinach leaf. Roll the wrapper and seal the edges with water. In a pan over medium high heat, add the vegetable oil. Cook the rolls until golden brown. Drain in paper towels. Divide cauliflower rice into 6 food containers. Add 3 cheesy spinach rolls in each food container. Toss cucumber and tomato in olive oil and vinegar. Place the cucumber tomato relish beside the rolls. Seal and reheat in the microwave when ready to serve.

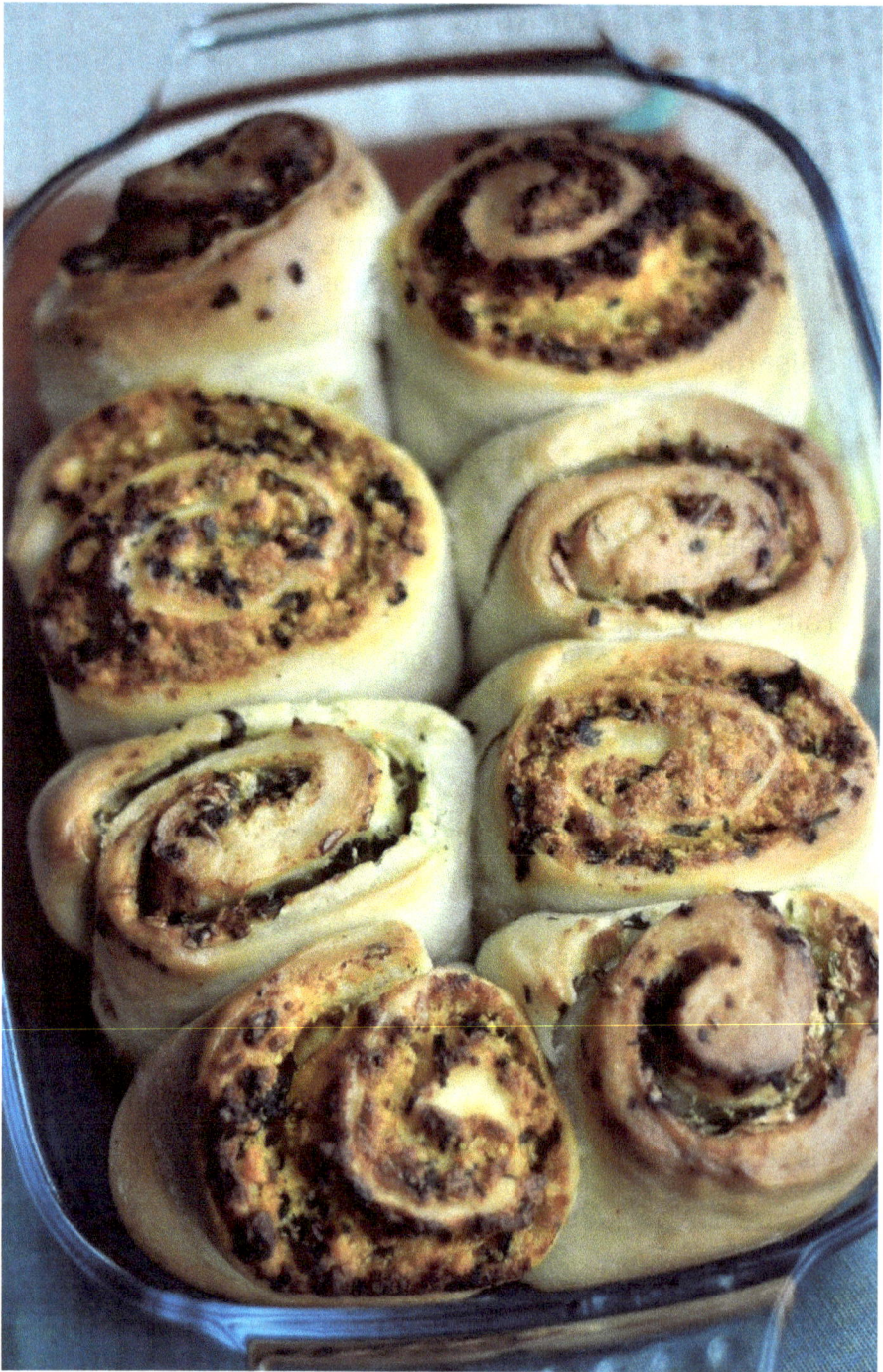

Superfood Buddha Bowl

Preparation Time: 10 minutes Cooking Time: 10 minutes Servings: 4

Ingredients:

8 oz. microwavable quinoa 2 tablespoons lemon juice ½ cup hummus Water 5 oz. baby kale 8 oz. cooked baby beets, sliced 1 cup frozen shelled edamame (thawed) ¼ cup sunflower seeds, toasted 1 avocado, sliced 1 cup pecans 2 tablespoons flaxseeds

Direction

Cook quinoa according to directions in the packaging. Set aside and let cool. In a bowl, mix the lemon juice and hummus. Add water to achieve desired consistency. Divide mixture into 4 condiment containers. Cover containers with lids and put in the refrigerator. Divide the baby kale into 4 food containers with lids. Top with quinoa, beets, edamame and sunflower seeds. Store in the refrigerator until ready to serve. Before serving add avocado slices and hummus dressing.

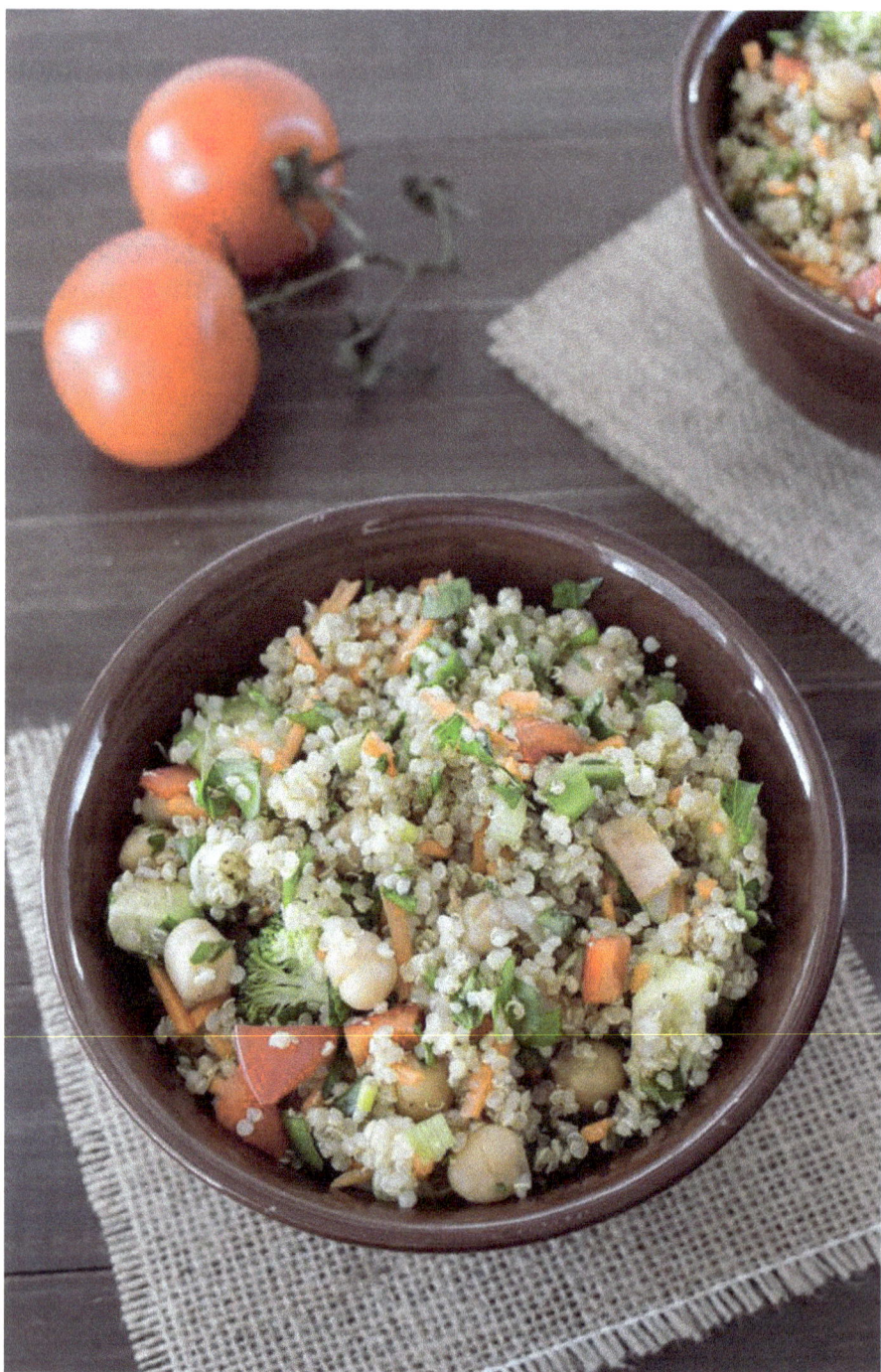

Super-Delicious Vegan Gravy

Preparation time: 10 minutes Cooking time: 40 minutesServings: 4.

Ingredients:

1 cup chopped mushrooms 3 tbsp. olive oil 3 chopped sage leaves 1 tsp. white wine 1 tsp. thyme 4 tbsp. vegan butter 3 tbsp. flour ¾ cup vegetable broth salt and pepper to taste

Directions:

Begin by heating together the mushrooms, the oil, the salt, and the herbs in a skillet. Cook the mushrooms for five minutes. Next, add the vinegar. Stir well for five minutes. Next, turn the heat to low, and add the flour and the butter. Stir well until you've creted a sort of paste. Add the vegetable broth, next, to create a smooth mixture. Turn the heat up to high once more, and stir until you've created a gravy. If your gravy is too thick, you can add a bit of soymilk to reach your consistency. Enjoy!

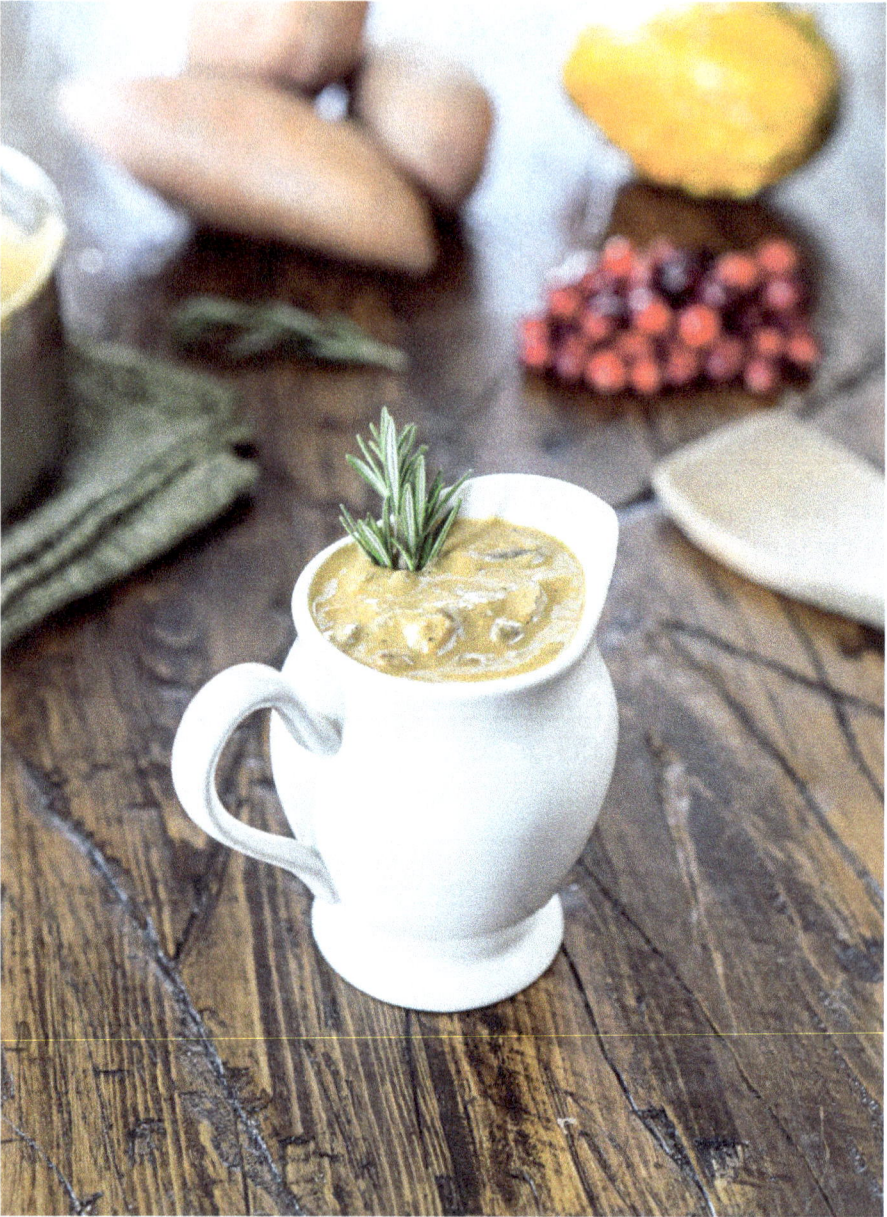

www.ingramcontent.com/pod-product-compliance
Lightning Source LLC
Chambersburg PA
CBHW050752030426
42336CB00012B/1789